BACK IN ACTION

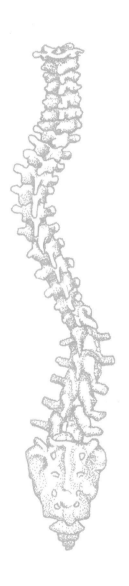

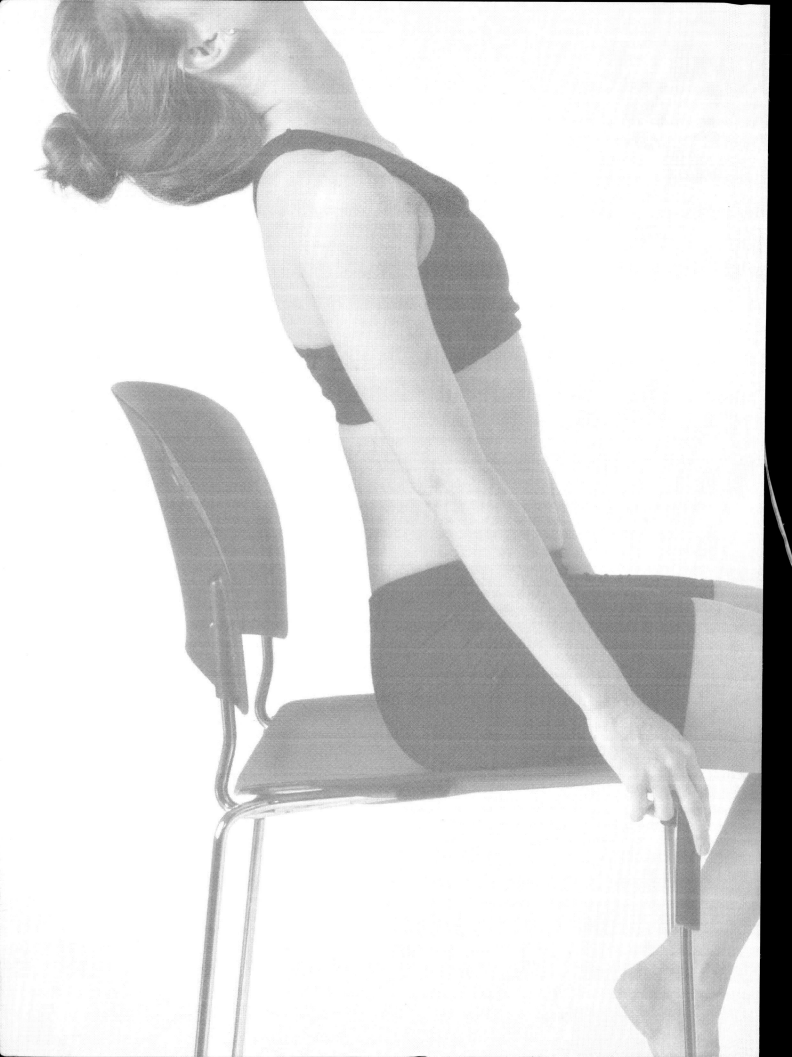

BACK IN ACTION

HEALING BACK PAIN THROUGH MOVEMENT

Scott G. Duke, DC, DACBSP, CSCS.

Chiropractic Sports Physician

Certified Strength and Conditioning Specialist

TIPS Technical Publishing, Inc.

Carrboro, North Carolina

Back in Action

ISBN 978-1-890586-32-4
eISBN 978-1-890586-33-1

Library of Congress Cataloging-in-Publication Data
Duke, Scott G.
  Back in action : healing back pain through movement / Scott G. Duke, DC, DACBSP, CSCS, Chiropractic Sports Physician, Certified Strength and Conditioning Specialist.
    pages cm
  Includes bibliographical references and index.
  ISBN 978-1-890586-32-4 (ISBN) -- ISBN 978-1-890586-33-1 (eISBN)
  1. Backache--Alternative treatment. 2. Back--Wounds and injuries. 3. Back exercises. I. Title.
  RD771.B217D84 2014
  617.5'64--dc23
                    2013040340

TIPS Technical Publishing, Inc.
108 E. Main Street, Suite 4
Carrboro, NC 27510
919-933-2629
www.technicalpublishing.com

Development editing by Karen Kelly
Book Design and ebook conversion by Robert Kern
Composition by Dale Koontz
Cover by Steven Klapow
Photography by Devvon Simpson
Videography by Chase Gordon
Diagrams by Kathy Telfer

Fot the millions of people who suffer needlessly from back pain

"The doctor of the future will give no medicine but will interest his patients in the care of the human frame, in diet, and in the cause and prevention of disease."

—Thomas Edison, Inventor

Notice to Readers

This publication contains the opinions and ideas of its author. It is intended to provide helpful and informative material on the subjects addressed in the publication. It is sold with the understanding that the author and publisher are not engaged in rendering medical, health, or any other kind of personal professional services in the book. The reader should consult his or her medical, health or other competent professional before adopting any of the suggestions in this book or drawing inferences from it.

The author and publisher specifically disclaim all responsibility for any liability, loss or risk, personal or otherwise, which is incurred as a consequence, directly or indirectly, of the use and application of any of the contents of this book.

CONTENTS

PREFACE

Freedom From Pain is in Your Hands

"Should I use ice or heat?"

"What is a disc?"

"Is bed rest the right thing to do?"

"Should I bend forward or backward?"

"Are sit-ups good for me?"

"Don't sit, don't stand, and don't lay down."

"It hurts to cough and sneeze…even laugh."

"I'm pregnant and have back pain. What do I do?"

"Do I need spine surgery?"

"My child has back pain. Should I be worried?"

"Should I wear a back support belt?"

"Are standing toe touches harmful?"

"My doctor said it's in my head."

These are things I hear on a daily basis. Over the past 25 years, after exhaustive clinical and biomedical research dedicated to the lower back, the number of back injuries has not declined. The delivery of medical services has increased and now most of the research is dedicated to developing ways to make those of you who suffer from back pain more comfortable.

Back pain is not a mystery; there are specific reasons why your back hurts and why back injuries occur. I'm here to shed light on low back pain and to help you understand why it happens, how you can heal it, and how to make sure you do not mismanage or exacerbate your condition ever again.

Many doctors reinforce the idea in patients' minds that their backs are ruined, degenerated, and fragile. I'm here to aid your awareness about back pain, and show you how you can benefit from a self-restorative process. You can cure yourself of back pain once you have the proper information and learn how to release your own potential to heal. I've heard over and over how a patient's lower back pain failed to respond to conventional treatments and rehabilitation approaches, how patients are accused by their doctors, therapists, and insurance carriers of not trying hard enough or being mentally tough. Unfortunately, the truth is that medical management has simply reached the end of its knowledge base and that's where the failure lies—not within you. *Back in Action* is your guide to self-care and self-healing.

Acknowledgements

To Penny, whom I love in a special way that the written word could never fully express; to Aaron & Chase, who kept the TV off so I could concentrate; and to LuLu, for not being upset when I failed my HS English regents…twice!

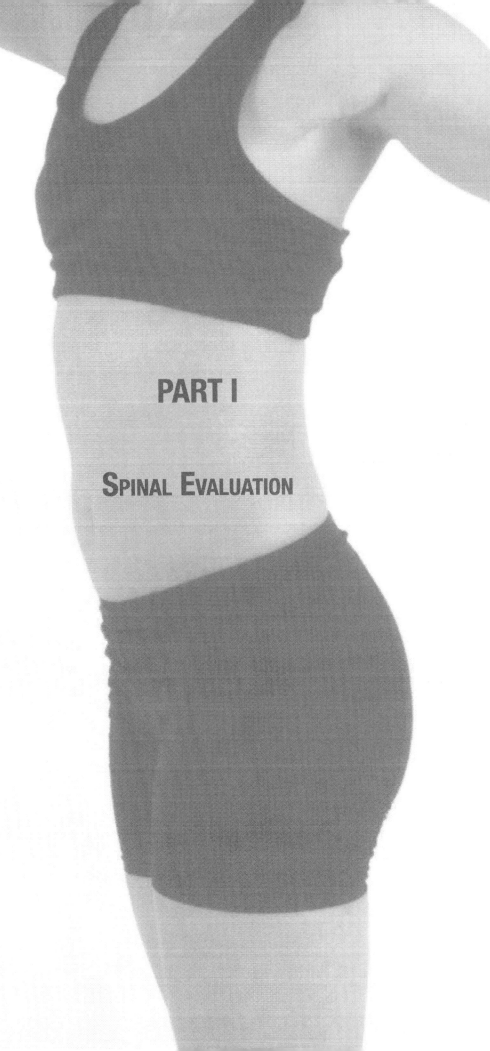

PART I

SPINAL EVALUATION

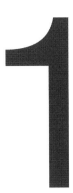

1

OUR FIRST CONSULTATION

Oh, the powers of nature! She knows what we
need, and the doctors know nothing.

—BENVENUTO CELLINI

"HI, I'M DR. DUKE and welcome to my office. I'm sorry you are so uncomfortable, but I'm sure I'll be able to help you." This is how I generally start all of my conversations with patients. When it comes to back pain, patients need to know that there is help as well as a way to feel better, and, as a physician, I need to put them at ease. I know I can help because, generally, the histories of the people who come to see me are similar and their stories are often the same, including tales of failed treatments, inadequate evaluations, over-diagnostic testing, and unsuccessful attempts to diagnose. Most of the time, as a physician who specializes in lower back pain, I can tell what's wrong with a patient just from their history, including what actions they took in the past to help resolve their condition, such as what worked, what didn't, who they saw, what medicines were prescribed, and the order of back pain events. I take as much time as needed to help them organize their thoughts, because trying to treat lower back pain can be very complicated and past events become blurred and challenging to recall. The longer you wait to see a doctor, or the more doctors you see, the more complicated things become. Essentially, too many chefs are in the kitchen! I usually ask my patients a series of questions that help me design an examination and create a treatment plan specifically geared for them.

Most of the time, I find that a patient was previously mismanaged, not on purpose, but simply because back pain is so challenging to resolve. Generally, I see the same treatment mistakes: a patient is given strength exercises when they need stretches, told to use heat when they need ice, or instructed to take rest when they need to be active. The list goes on and on. By the time they make it to my office, they have already seen a gamut of doctors. These patients have probably been given all the right remedies, but because the remedies may have been dispensed in the wrong order, the patient feels deflated and defeated, believing nothing will work. Chiropractors, unfortunately, are usually the last stop, a last ditch effort. It's really too bad, in my opinion. People should consider chiropractors as a first line of defense because we are, in fact, the primary physicians for back care and pain.

As a chiropractic sports physician, I can save your back. Chiropractors are spinal health care experts who have the ability to improve function in the neuro-muscular-skeletal system, as well as overall health, well-being and quality of life. We have a tradition of effectiveness and patient satisfaction without the use of drugs or surgery. As expertly qualified providers of spinal manipulation, many soft-tissue massage treatments, and therapeutic exercise instruction, we collaborate with other health professionals and emphasize the self-healing powers of the individual and encourage patient independence.

Throughout this text you will find an endless supply of effective ways to help heal your back pain, supported and documented by evidence-based research and deciphered for your general use. You will learn effective ways to self manage when injured, specific action sequences and movements to relieve stiffness and soreness, exercises which are harmful to the spine (and possibly keeping you injured), postures to avoid, and a plethora of self-help advice to use when suffering an acute back attack.

Essentially this book will be your back pain resource—your personal Madison Ave. spine care specialist. I designed this book so you feel as if you are one-on-one with your doctor—receiving all the attention you rightfully deserve.

I look forward to helping you. Your in great hands.

Best in health,
Dr. Duke

2

THE STRAW THAT BROKE THE CAMEL'S BACK

In health there is freedom. Health is the first of all liberties.
—Henri-Frederic Amiel, 1828–1881

THE ALARM GOES OFF early in the morning. After rolling out of bed and shuffling to the bathroom, you bend forward to pick a towel up from the floor and wham! Your back goes out. You try to straighten up but you can't. You're bent and tilted to one side, and the pain is so intense that you can't even take a deep breath. You close your eyes and tell yourself to stay calm. A few minutes pass and you try to move, but feel another zing in your back, dropping you to the floor. Writhing around on the cold tile, you wonder how this could have happened. All you did was try to pick up a towel!

I hear some version of this story almost every day. Most patients tell me, "Doc, all I did was bend over to put on my shoe," or "I was just brushing my teeth." "I woke up with it!" "All I did was sneeze!" Get the picture? You're not the only one to have a back attack! You probably had warning signs before you were immobilized, such as back soreness, occasional twinges and spasms, or a general feeling of tightness that you thought would go away on their own. Unfortunately, those dull aches and stabbing pains lead to misery and disability for millions of sufferers. Often, people are so happy when their back pain finally lessens that they immediately think they're cured and turn their attention elsewhere. That's part of the problem.

You might have thought your back attack was a fluke because it happened while you were doing something you've done thousands of times before, like picking up a towel off the bathroom floor. Don't adopt the standard attitude of, "Okay, I hurt my back so I'll just rest it until the pain goes away." The pain is going to return and next time it will be even more intense. This cycle will continue until you find yourself sitting in a doctor's office explaining that the so-called on-and-off back pain has been occurring for some time now with difficulty narrowing down when it all began.

Here are the facts. Once you injure your back, you're likely to have episodic back pain for up to two years. You'll probably have relapses during the first year, each lasting longer and with greater intensity than the last. During these episodes, you may be pain-free after about two weeks' time. However, if your back pain starts to linger more than 30 days or so, research tells us that you will continue to have on-and-off low back symptoms for another one to five years.

At this point, not only is your back pain here, it's here to stay.

Until now, that is. My clinical experience tells me that mismanagement is the primary reason so many people suffer from episodic low back pain. Patients visit doctor after doctor, trying to find the answers to their back pain. They finally end up at a specialist's office, via a friend's recommendation, only to sadly find no new advice or miracle medication to cure their ailments. Instead, they learn that there are as many doctors as there are answers to the question "How do I treat my back pain?" Patients will hear advise like this:

- Use ice
- Apply heat
- Try muscle relaxers
- Try bed rest
- Stay active
- Sleep on your stomach

- Take anti-inflammatories
- Don't stretch
- Strengthen your back
- Just pull your knees to your chest, that'll do it.
- Try yoga

Ridiculous, isn't it? Not to mention completely frustrating and many times just plain wrong.

When conventional medicine proves unhelpful, sufferers finally step out of the box and seek help from alternative medical providers. In 2009, Harvard University conducted a national survey and found that 50% of all patients with back pain who consulted with alternative medical providers did so in secret and without seeking advice from their primary medical doctors. How crazy is it that patients are so frustrated with the care they've received that they are afraid to fess up to seeing an alternative provider because they thought their doctors wouldn't approve?

The good news is that real answers are out there. Proven research, a collaborated effort from multi-disciplinary medical and chiropractic panels from around the world, and guidelines developed specifically to improve patient outcome are available to help you treat low back pain. However, these resources are so complicated, detailed, and difficult to decipher that most doctors can't keep up.

I wrote this book to simplify this information and demystify one of medicine's most frustrating conditions, and to assure you that there is no shame in educating yourself about your health or seeking the guidance of an alternative health provider. I've consolidated the most advanced, up-to-date medical research and combined it with over 22 years of clinical experience, with nearly 200,000 successful spinal treatments, to put an end to this epidemic of mismanagement, poor communication, and ongoing pain.

I've created a dynamic, "Back in Action" sequence of spinal exercises that promote movement without the associated risk of injury. Think of these exercises as ways to prepare your body for motion. They are safe exercises that lubricate the joints, reduce inflammation, wake up muscles and tendons, and activate and protect your spine.

I also wrote this book so you don't have to immediately rush to the doctor's office the next time your back goes out, and so you won't have to simply take the "wait and hope" approach for your back pain to disappear. *Back in Action* should be a resource for you and, if you wish, for your doctor as well—not to mention your masseuse, personal trainer, physical therapist, wellness coach, and everyone that is involved with back pain. Also, anyone involved in health care should own this book. It a manual which teaches how to prevent back pain. It's intended to be a guide that explains and demonstrates precisely what to do from day one, whether your back is in the acute or chronic stage of pain.

Most "back attacks" are expressions of underlying chronic problems. Even if you've had it for years, here's your opportunity to start over successfully and put an end to this condition. So, pull yourself together and follow my advice.

Let me be clear—there is no single, miraculous exercise, injection, medication, or surgery to fix low back pain. However, there are scientifically proven exercise techniques and common modifications of daily activities that, when properly executed, will help heal low back pain and reduce the likelihood of recurrent symptoms.

As you begin to educate yourself about your back pain, consider yourself a patient in one of the world's finest spine care facilities, ready to receive all of this amazing information for the price of less than an insurance copayment. Forget about how it all began and start to focus on how to end it. Just follow my "keep it simple and safe" approach and consider this a physician's desk reference designed for you, my patient. I look forward to saving you from unnecessary trips to the doctor's office, medical bills, insurance premiums, and lost time from work and family. It's a journey, and we're in it together. Let's get started.

Movements That Destroy the Spine

In order to heal the spine, one must first stop maintaining its injuries. I'll start by revealing exercises which (although commonly prescribed to help people with lower back pain) are, unfortunately, horrible for the spine. So if you perform any of the below movements, STOP IMMEDIATELY. You are essentially keeping your spine injured and it will never heal.

Bad and Worse

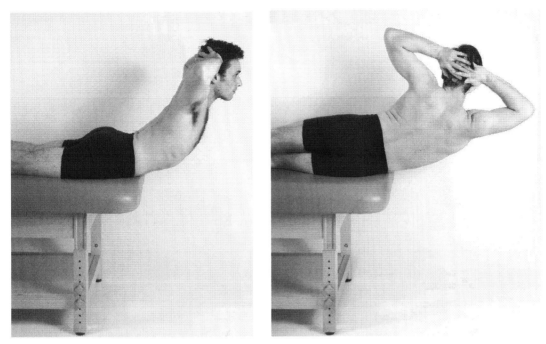

Back extensions (left) place nearly 900 pounds of compression per repetition on the lower back. Roman chair back bends (right) shear the spinal discs.

Horrible and Destructive

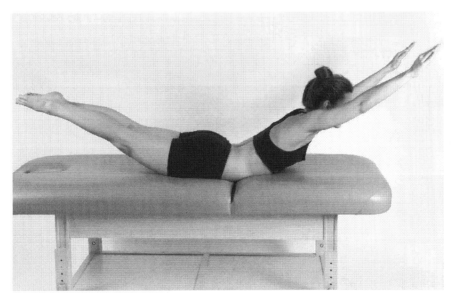

"Superman" exercises place nearly 1,400 pounds of compression per repetition on the lower back.

It hurts me just to look at these exercises. The damage people do to their backs when performing these movements is incredible. The biomechanics of these motions are horribly destructive to your spine. There is a limit for low back compression—675 lbs. Sounds like a lot doesn't it? Repeated loading above this level is linked with high rates of low back injuries. Simply put, the spinal tissues can't handle the load when they're repeatedly forced to handle above 675 lbs.

Leg lifts, back extensions, and the superman are exercises that place enormous loads on the spinal joints. It may not happen at first, but over time your spinal joints will wear out, causing cartilage to become grainy like sand, discs to degenerate, and arthritis to set in. Over time, the spine weakens, which is why most people injure their lower backs following a movement they've performed hundreds or thousands of times before. Literally, that one movement becomes the straw that breaks the camel's back.

I need you to understand why these and other movements are horrible for the spine. This way, the next time you hire a trainer or therapist, you can question their ability if they try to sell you on these exercises. I've trained hundreds, if not thousands, of personal trainers throughout my career in New York City on injury prevention. I can assure you, if someone you know is prescribing these activities, they're giving you a prescription for back pain.

While I'm sure the following exercises are not performed with the purpose of doing damage, most attempts at physical therapy for the back include the common use of the exercises described in this section. These exercises are also often recommended by personal trainers and commonly performed in a health club setting to strengthen your core. I'll also review other exercises commonly done at the gym and at home later in the book.

I'm truly sick over the misuse of the word "core." It has been wrongly applied by so many people for so many different things that it has essentially lost its meaning. Unfortunately, these exercises create back pain and set up the spine for injury. Don't do them. Each crunch compresses the low back with approximately 675 lbs. of pressure. This is the equivalent to NIOSH (The National Institute of Occupational Safety and Health) limits for safe low back compression. Repetitive loads of this amount increase the likelihood of back injury and will, over time, cause spinal back failure. Back arching, like the Roman chair, produces 900–1,000 lbs. of compression and the superman results in nearly 1,400 lbs. of compression with each repetition.

My question is this: why perform these exercises at all? There are better ways to challenge the abdominal and low back muscles, and I will review my prescribed core endurance exercises in the next section. One of the best ways to maximize the benefits of exercise is to really understand the way your muscles work when using them. I will briefly teach you the basics, as I do for all of my patients.

Muscles 101

PSOAS (pronounced "soas") is a giant hip flexor muscle that connects your hip to the front of your low back by attaching itself to every vertebra from T12 to L4 with the exception of L5.

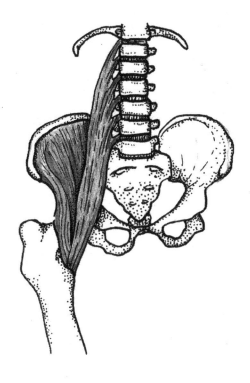

Diagram 1: Psoas (hip flexor) muscle

This muscle is commonly used when performing crunches, sit-ups, and leg lifts. People think they are training their abs, but in reality, they're just over working their hip flexors to the point where the psoas becomes preferentially recruited in lieu of the abdominal wall. So, the abs become flabby and weak as the psoas becomes stronger, tighter, and shorter.

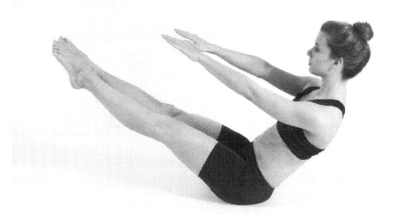

Leg lifts over develop the hip flexors, weaken the
abdominal wall and shear the lower spine.

As this muscle shortens, because of its orientation to the spine, it tugs the spine forward, literally jamming the low back together, like a loaded spring, causing compression to the lumbar facet joints. These joints are loaded with pain-sensitive nerve endings. When jammed up, they create muscle spasms, reduce oxygenated blood flow, and become responsible for most early degenerative arthritic changes that occur in the low back.

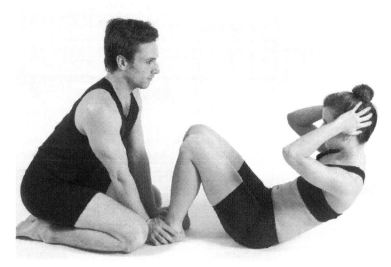

Sit-ups and crunches work the hip flexor, not the abs.

Oblique Crunches

This exercise creates torque on your spine. Flattening the low back while twisting is a recipe for disaster. This motion is perfect for rupturing a low back disc, as it places it in a vulnerable posture that weakens the protective character of the spinal joints.

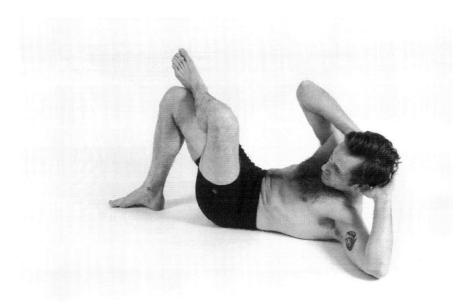

Oblique crunches can rupture lower back disks.

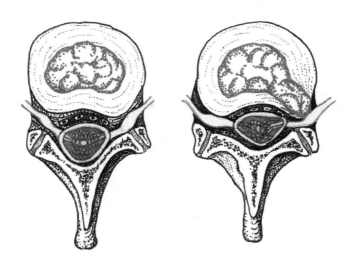

Diagram 2: Normal disc (left). Herniated disc pinching a nerve (right).

Standing Side Bends and Roman Chair—Side Bends

These exercises do not train your abdomen at all. Rather, these motions train a postural muscle called the Quadratus Lumborum (QL). This muscle is a hip hiker, and it connects your ribs and diaphragm to your pelvis while also attaching to the side of your spine. This muscle is a workhorse designed to anchor and stabilize your spine. When it's trained via motion, it creates a horribly detrimental shearing force that hikes your hip up, giving you a functional short leg. This short leg is apparent with stance, walking, and running: it strains your spine with every step you take. This muscle is not meant to move your spine. It's meant to stabilize it, not shear it.

When people perform these ridiculous exercises the muscle begins to become short and tight. Eventually, this muscle locks your spine in this awkward posture, creating an environment that prematurely wears out your spine and herniates your discs.

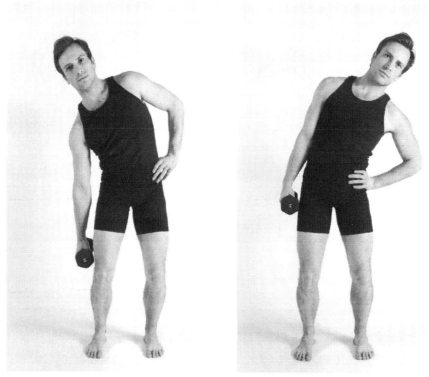

Standing side bends

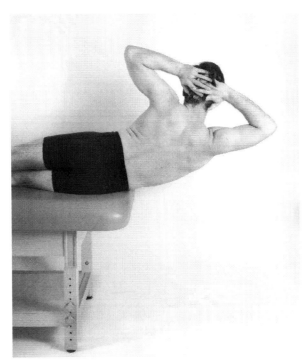

Roman chair side bends

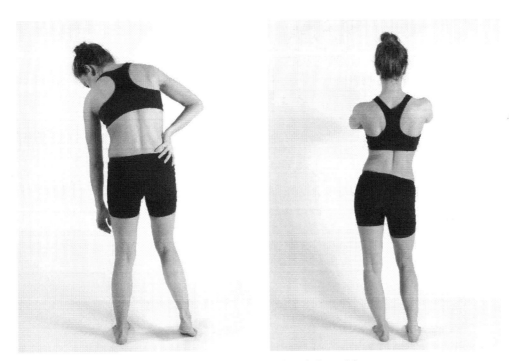

Side bends contribute to these back breaking postures.

Quadriceps

Known as your quad or thigh muscle, it is also a hip flexor. It attaches the top crest of your pelvis to your kneecap by running the entire length of your thigh. It is a two-joint muscle, meaning it crosses your hip joint and your knee joint. When short and tight, this muscle stoops your low back forward and causes a swayback posture.

Most people try to stretch this muscle by standing upright and pulling their heel to their buttock. However, this stretch is essentially useless as it does not target the origin of the muscle located at the top of the pelvis and puts tremendous and harmful strain on the kneecap.

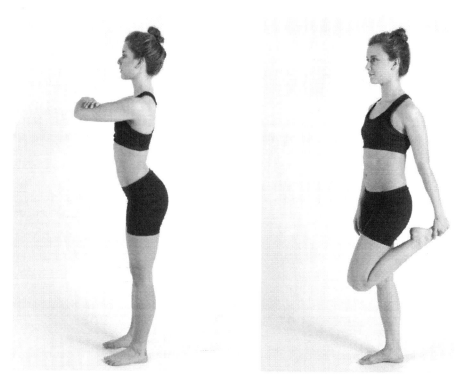

Sway back posture from tight quadriceps (left). Quad stretch which puts harmful strain on the kneecap (right).

Since you are only stretching the muscle at the kneecap, the top part remains short and tight, consequently locking the pelvis forward. This posture may also occur on just half of your pelvis, causing a pelvic distortion where half is rotated forward and half is rotated backward, further distorting your posture and setting you up for future back attacks.

Any active person who adopts a distorted pelvis will be more vulnerable to lower back injury, even if they feel they are in excellent shape. This is why back attacks happen to people who perform movements they have done thousands of times. Then one day, seemingly spontaneously, this same motion throws out their back!

Hamstrings

This muscle attaches from your "sit-bone," the ischial tuberosity, and runs down the back of your thigh and under your calf. It also runs beneath the buttock and attaches via tendons and fasciae to your lower back. When short and tight, this muscle flattens the low back and takes away its natural curve. Clinically, patients with a flat back posture generally have a variety of low back problems, such as spinal stenosis (a clogging of the spinal canal diameter) which leads to a stooped posture distortion.

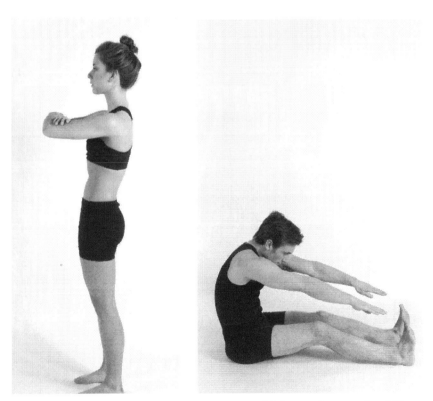

Tight hamstrings create a flat back posture which weakens spinal ligaments.

Piriformis

This muscle is a hip rotator, attaching your outer hip to the sacrum. The sacrum is the triangular bone above your coccyx and is considered the base of your spine. It is also known as S1 or the Sacro-Iliac Joint. When short and tight, this muscle will turn your leg outward, resulting in a posture that moves the muscle closer to the sciatic nerve.

Eventually, this muscle may rip or strain, causing inflammation and direct compression on your sciatic nerve—a condition commonly known as piriformis syndrome. Patients suffering from this condition feel as if someone stabbed a hot poker in their buttock which shoots electrical signals down the back of their thighs into the bottom of their feet.

Lastly, because the muscle attaches to the sacrum, it may pull and tug the joint, creating sacroiliac instability or SI Joint Dysfunction.

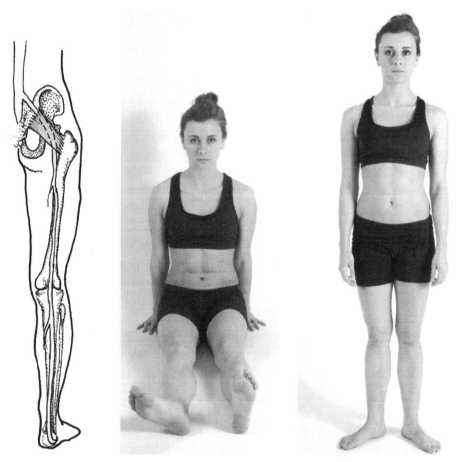

Diagram 3: Sciatic nerve running through piriformis muscle (left).
Tight piriformis muscles effect on posture (center and right).

Glute Medius

This muscle is located on the side of the butt, above your hipbone, and helps keep the pelvis level.

When standing on one leg and holding your balance, this muscle is activated. When short, tight, and weak, it may be slow to engage, causing the unsupported side to drop down.

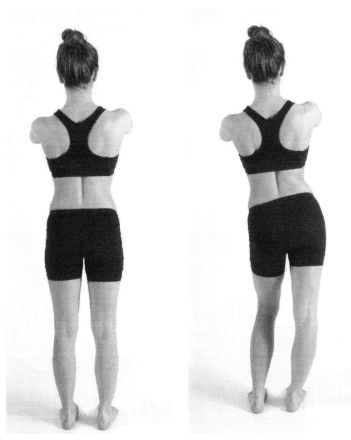

The glute medius muscle helps keep your pelvis level.

This is characteristic of a lurched gait or someone with a barely noticeable limp. It becomes most apparent with walking and running and is horribly detrimental to the spine. By the time a weakness is detected, the body has usually adapted to the abnormal motion, which feels normal to the person with low back pain. This issue is generally associated with a degenerative hip and hip replacement surgery.

Spinal Erectors

This is not one muscle but several groups of muscles that run the entire length of your torso, from the base of your skull to the tip of your coccyx.

The function of the spinal erectors is to keep your spine erect and upright. When deconditioned, they cannot support the spine. Most people, with or without low back pain, feel tight and sore in this area and consequently try to stretch it out.

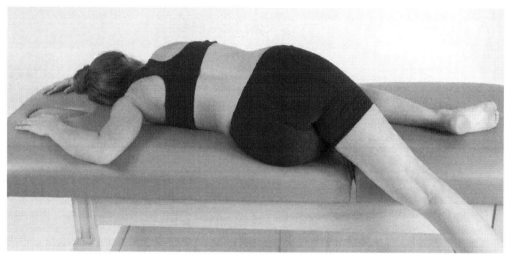

Spinal twist stretch: a good stretch for the spinal erector muscle group.

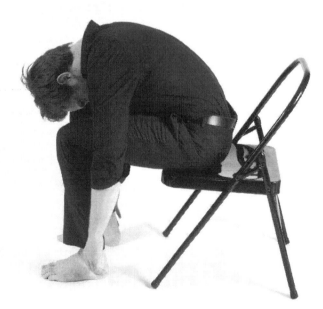

Chair stretch: a bad stretch for the spinal erector muscle group.

The chair stretch above is a mistake. Generally, these muscles are weak and require strengthening to help stabilize the spine. When you stretch them out, you create further instability and place an excessive load on the lower back that can lead to joint failure. For those of you who have mistakenly stretched out these muscles over the years, let's turn our attention on how to safely normalize their length and take that unwanted tension off your spine.

The Right Movements for Everyday Living

Now that you know your anatomy and what movements are bad for your back, let's learn ways to lift, bend, stoop, and carry properly. Here's a basic primer on how to protect your spine while living a normal life.

Slips and Falls

We can't help it—we trip, we fall… it happens. However, people with low back trouble show a delay in torso muscle core activation during sudden events like these. Their back problem impairs the ability of the spine to attain a protective state when needed. The lack of a protective state has to do with fatigue and a lack of endurance in your low back muscles. The core exercises prescribed in this book emphasize endurance and using pain as your guide. Doing so will train your spine to develop a protective mechanism that will go into action when necessary.

Heavy Lifting

Maintaining an arch in the lower back while lifting heavy objects ensures a high tolerance of the spinal joints to withstand compression. Thus, it reduces—and in some cases eliminates—the risk of ligament, disc, and muscle damage (as compared to a flexed and rounded lower back, which increases these risks).

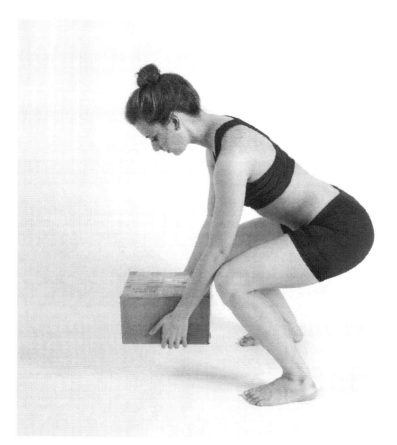

Proper form for heavy lifting—maintaining an arch in lower back.

The challenge here is that it is physiologically more difficult and expends more energy to squat and lunge versus stooping so that people get hurt because they take the seemingly easy way out when lifting. Consider Olympic weight lifters. They lock their spine with a natural arch, enabling them to lift enormous loads while limiting the spinal load.

Remember, most disc herniations happen as a result of repeated low back flexion or a rounded lower back posture. Avoidance of this posture while lifting minimizes the cumulative effect that often results in lower back injury. Furthermore, the emphasis should be to place the load as close to your body as possible when lifting.

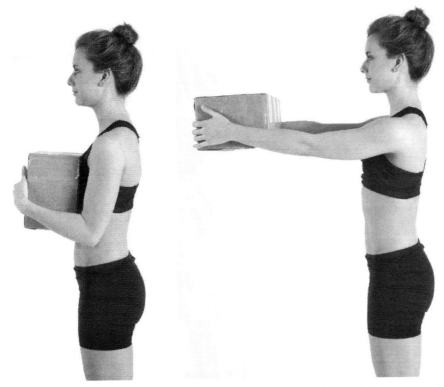

When lifting keep object close to the body to reduce lower back stress. Image on left shows proper form while image on right shows poor form.

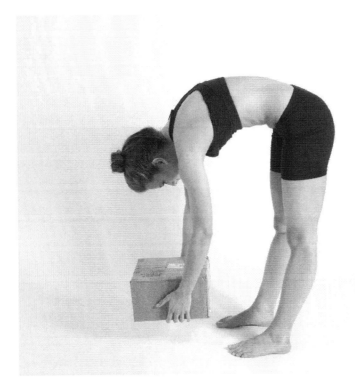

Lifting with a rounded lower back and straight legs can rupture a spinal disc.

Light Lifting

For repeated lifting of light objects, like pencils, paper, toys, and tissues, use the golfer's lift to minimize low back damage. The leg is cantilevered behind and rotated about the hip with the arm forward for balance.

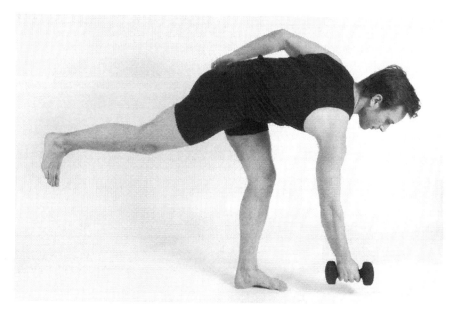

Use the golfer's lift for light loads.

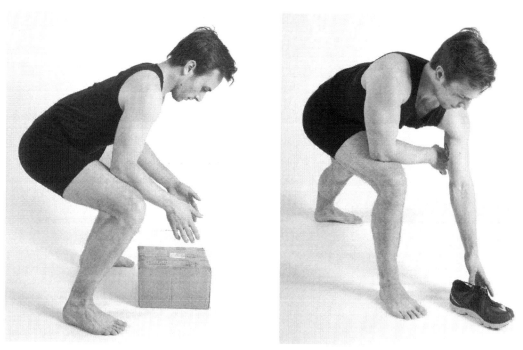

Proper lifting techniques for heavy (left) and light (right) objects.

Most people still adhere to the misguided old school instructions to bend at the knees and squat. The golfer's lift conserves muscle and joint energy, works on balance, and places little demand on the knees when lifting light objects. If you are really stiff in the morning, place both hands on your thighs and slowly squat down while placing most of your weight onto your arms and thighs instead of on your low back. This will help alleviate most low back pressure.

Pushing and Pulling

When pushing or pulling, most people do so diagonally through their shoulders. This movement creates a large force vector, which is especially damaging to the spine. Instead, stand closer to the object and push/pull directly in front of you. Try to tighten your abdomen as well. This spares the spine from unnecessary twisting and torque. Use this posture with any activity, from shoveling and sweeping to opening and closing doors.

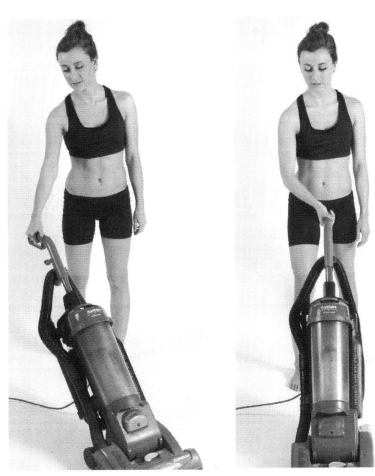

Improper pushing diagonally with shoulders (left).
Proper pushing directly in front of you (right).

Twisting

One way to injure your back is to twist your spine while bending forward, such as when you take luggage from a car trunk. Luckily, the spine has protective facet joints. They stop rotation well before the elastic limits of the discs are reached. However, twisting while bending forward takes out all the protection of these facet joints and promotes a high risk of disc injury. Instead, slowly shimmy the object to a point where it's as close to your chest as possible, maintain a natural curve in the low back to prevent a stooped posture, and then squat and lift.

Strolling

Walking slowly increases low back pain. When you walk in a museum, shopping mall, or a local street fair, we call this "mall strolling pace." It's a slow pace, where you apply nearly 2.5 times your body weight in compression with every step. However, when you walk faster, say at a brisk walk greater than 3 mph, you can generally cover a distance of one mile in 20 minutes. It's a pace that almost forces you to swing your arms, and in doing so, you create a movement of the spine known as oscillation, a general rhythmic motion in which you reduce spinal compression. Brisk walking has shown to be strongly associated with successful recovery in low back pain.

Sitting

Following 20 minutes of sitting, spinal ligaments soften and elongate. Posture is no longer in check due to this lack of stability. The disc gel begins to migrate backwards, meaning that the protective cartilage barriers that surround the disc are weakened. If you work at a desk and bend forward to pick a pencil up from the floor, you can injure your back and herniate a disc. It takes roughly two minutes of standing and arching backwards to regain about 50% of the protective joint stiffening caused by just 20 minutes of sitting or slouching. It can take about 30 minutes of standing to regain the full protection following a seated posture.

I generally recommend that you don't immediately sit when you wake up in the morning. Look at the posture shown next. Of course your back hurts. All the ligaments are stretched out, your discs are leaking fluid backwards, and if you already have a herniated disc, sitting early in the morning will absolutely kill your back. Instead, stand for the first 30 minutes of the day. This will allow enough time for the spine to reset back to normal and avoid additional strain.

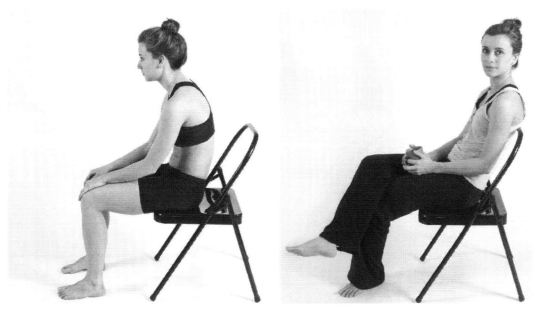

Sitting in the morning causes spinal ligaments to soften and elongate, leading to back injuries and herniated discs.

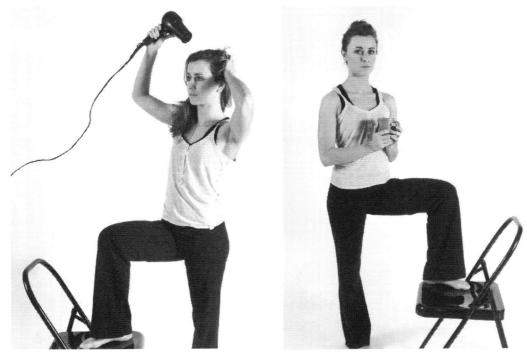

Standing for 30 minutes in the morning resets the spine to normal.

Sitting and Disc Herniations

Experts have seen a link between seated posture and herniated discs since the 1970s. The fact is, there is no ideal seated posture. Rather, a variable one is recommended—in other words, your next posture is your best posture. The ideal seated posture is a continually changing one, which prevents the spine structure from accumulating too much stress. A sitting position that changes the spinal load frequently minimizes the risk of any single ligament, muscle, or disc from accumulating a continuous load that can injure it. Use ergonomic chairs and learn how to adjust the seat height, angles, and rotation, and use them frequently throughout the day.

Get out of your chair about once an hour. There's no substitute for standing upright after sitting. Just stand up and arch backwards. Perform the *Back in Action* exercises prescribed in this book. This will keep your joints limber and your muscles activated in an attempt to prevent microtrauma from the accumulated loads of sitting still.

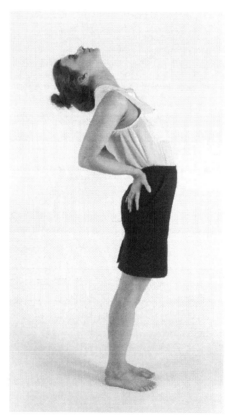

To stretch out after sitting, simply stand up and arch backwards.

Lastly, never, ever bend forward after sitting for awhile. The aches you feel are stretched out ligaments and muscles. If you feel the urge to stretch out your low back, think the opposite and arch backwards. Bending forward while sitting or immediately after is the most vulnerable time for your spine—a back attack just waiting to happen.

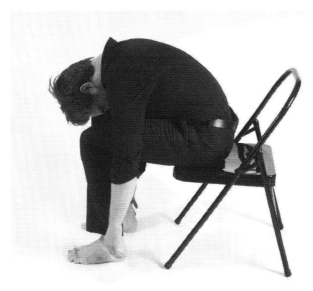

Never stretch out the back by bending forward following sitting!

Stoop Posture and Back Pain

When the back stoops forward, your low back muscles shut down. The ligaments are recruited to stabilize the spine. This is normal; it's called the Flexion-Relaxation Response. Experts estimate that 225 lbs. of pressure are placed on the spine in a stooped posture and that this approaches the maximum compression the spine can handle before it buckles.

In a neutral posture (illustrated next), a lordotic C-shaped curve is adopted and the sheer spinal loads are reduced to about 45 lbs. So, by using your muscles to lock your back in a neutral posture, you reduce the spinal load by nearly 500% and also greatly reduce your chance of lower back injury.

> **Parents of newborns frequently injure their backs by carefully placing their infants up & down over the crib cage in a stooped posture— constantly straining their spines until one day *wham*, it buckles.**

How to Find Neutral

Finding neutral means finding a comfortable position for your spine some-where between being too arched and too flexed. Think of Goldilocks and the three bears; your neutral feels "just right." By finding that sweet spot, you ensure reduced spinal stress, which means less low back pain. Let's learn how. Place your hands on your back and stomach, arch and flatten a few times and find a comfortable in-between posture. That position is your personal neutral.

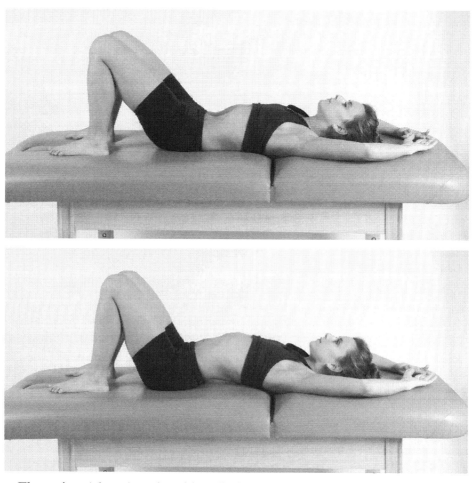

Flattening (above) and arching (below) to find neutral. Your personal neutral is the comfortable spot between these extremes.

Once you find neutral while lying on your back, try the same maneuvers while standing. Adding gravity makes this movement more challenging. However, it is very important to have body awareness in a standing posture.

Basically, the spine is much safer with a C-shaped curve versus a rounded and flexed posture. It's been shown that a rounded lower back posture is 40%

weaker and more vulnerable to injury than a neutral C-shaped lower back posture. Remember—neutral is best!

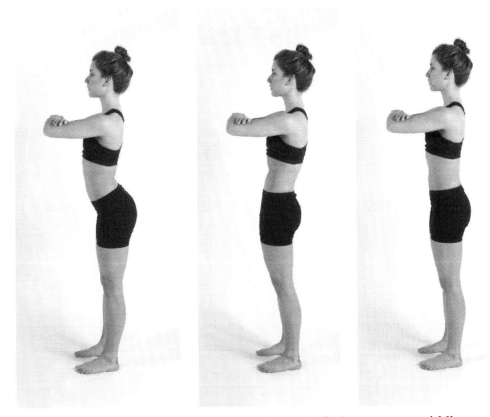

Find neutral from a standing position. Left shows sway, middle shows flat, and right shows neutral position.

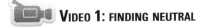 VIDEO 1: FINDING NEUTRAL

All-Day Habit: The Abdominal Brace

Our abdomens are composed of four different muscle groups, that, when activated in unison, create a hoop that wraps around our waist and back and is connected by tissue called fascia. If we train our abdominal muscles to remain active during our activities of daily living, we create an anatomical brace that protects our lower back. Unfortunately, most people don't know how to activate their abdominal brace during their normal activities. When they think of abdominal muscles, they think of sit-ups and crunches. Next is a photo of an inactive abdominal wall and a posture called abdominal hollowing. "Tuck your belly button inward" is commonly prescribed as a means to activate your abdomen: as you'll see, this is terrible for the spine.

Look at the two photos showing side views. The model is creating a flat back, probably the absolute worst posture anyone can have. It's a stance that is linked with spinal failure and buckling actions of the low back because it disables the protective forces of the low back erector muscles. Conventionally, patients with chronic lower back pain were given the hollowing exercise below to train the transverse abdominis, the deepest layer of the abdominal wall. This muscle has gotten a lot of attention in medical research, in part because it is involved in the belt-like containment of the abdomen, but mostly because the transverse abdominis has a delayed onset of activation in those with low back pain who are involved in a rapid activity.

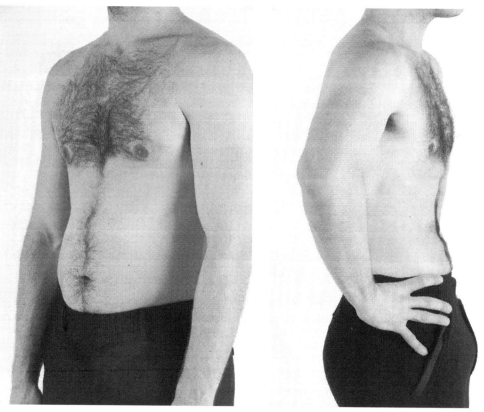

Inactive abdominal wall (left) and abdominal hollowing (right). Both postures offer little spinal protection.

The problem I have is that delayed onset means 10–30 milliseconds, or 1/10 of a second. I question whether it's really relevant during normal movements when we need our muscles to be continually active to ensure stability. The fact is, we have other abdominal muscles which can help stabilize the spine when used as a co-activation. This means opposing muscle groups located in the front and back of your torso, and opposing muscle groups located on the left and right flank fire and contract simultaneously, creating a corset of strength. This is opposed to what some old-fashioned-thinking exercise therapists might do, which is simply to focus on the transversus abdominus—just one muscle located deep in the abdominal wall. This muscle has too much attention paid to it in lieu of working on the entire corset that surrounds your torso. Paying attention to the transverse abdominus alone is a common error in spine rehabilitation.

Teaching someone to flatten their back is setting them up for spinal failure and chronic low back pain. Imagine hollowing your abdomen in an attempt to activate the transverse abdominus right before you lift or squat. This is a herniated disc just waiting to happen. The transverse abdominus is important to activate, but not at the expense of a flattened lower back.

The solution is to tighten all the layers of the abdomen at once, without changing our posture or holding our breath. Imagine that someone is going to punch you in the stomach. You probably just tightened all the abdominal muscles you could, and you are probably holding your breath as well. This is called intra-abdominal pressure (IAP). This elevated pressure enhances the stability of the spine. However, you can have adequate IAP without holding your breath. You need to practice breathing normally while simultaneously holding your abdominal muscles tight.

To brace properly, one needs to breathe normally while performing this movement. This is essential to help protect your spine from unguarded movements, which can harm and cause a buckling effect, damaging the joints, discs, and so on. You see, anatomically, we are all built with the same machinery. The problem is that as we get deconditioned, older, or injured, the machinery doesn't work as well. We need to retrain our corset. Think of it as a software update.

Abdominal bracing is an attempt to tighten all layers of the torso at once without changing your posture or breathing pattern. Try this: Stiffen your elbow by simultaneously tightening your biceps and triceps. Stiffen it so no one can straighten it out. Feel it? This is co-activation. You tightened the front and back at once, creating a brace. Bracing may be difficult at first; however, it's very important to master because it's a tool that can literally save your back from injury. At the end of any of the *Back in Action* routines described here, and once your spine is limber and lubricated, perform the abdominal brace to set it in place and stiffen your core, an action that will help stabilize your spine throughout the day. You can't perform this move enough. Practice bracing all day so that you become so adept at it that it eventually becomes natural to do with easy breathing. The goal is to brace a hundred times a day to help stiffen your spine 2–3 seconds at a time. Whatever you do, don't hollow your stomach and don't flatten your back. It reduces your base of stability.

Instead, engage all the muscles of your abdominal wall at once and maintain the natural curve in your low back, essentially bearing down as if you were constipated and couldn't have a bowel movement. Only don't hold your breath! Sorry for the blunt analogy, but I needed to get my point across. Better yet, pretend as if someone is about to punch you in the stomach and you tighten up all at once….this is an abdominal brace to protect your spine.

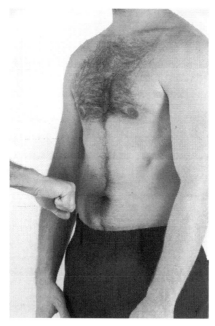

Abdominal brace to protect your spine

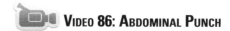 **Video 86: Abdominal Punch**

Here's how you do it:

1. Tighten your buttocks while seated and focus on the sensation of touching the seat.
2. Next, tighten and relax different muscles throughout your body, such as your arms, thighs, calves, neck, etc. This technique teaches you body awareness.
3. Now feel your abs and try to tighten and relax them. Look in the mirror if you need visual feedback.
4. Lastly, try bracing. Tighten your buttocks and abs at the same time, but don't hold your breath.

Practice the brace while sitting and standing. Then start practicing while reaching across a desk, pulling a door open, lifting a child, putting on shoes, and so on.

Abdominal bracing is like a low-back savings account; the more you invest (brace), the more low-back security you create. The more you attempt to brace your abs, the more natural it becomes. Before you know it, you're bracing without even realizing it. It becomes ingrained in your nervous system to occur naturally. Remember, most people injure their lower backs performing movements they've already done hundreds, if not thousands, of times.

By learning to brace before an action is performed, like opening a window, you protect your spine from trauma. It's when you don't brace while performing these daily tasks that you cause microtrauma which will wear out the spine (slowly tearing it apart) until finally—whack—your back buckles and you suffer a back injury.

Have fun. Brace all day. And, remember to never, ever hold your breath!

Activate Your Core

The following exercises teach your body to activate the core and stabilize the spine while in various postures. It's unreasonable to think that being on the floor is the only time to work on your core. You need to call upon it while standing, kneeling, and if you find yourself on all fours. Life is full of cracks in the sidewalk, potholes in the streets, uneven terrain on the grass or pathways, and it's completely unpredictable whether you're being active, playing with kids, or cleaning while on your hands and knees. The scenarios are commonplace. Learn to activate your abdominal corset in various postures. It's what we ask of our bodies in real life.

Abdominal Bracing Exercises

All 4's

While in the cat and cow posture, find neutral (the place between a swayed back and a flat back that feels comfortable) and tighten all of your abdominal muscles. Hold strong while focusing on breathing in and out fully and effortlessly.

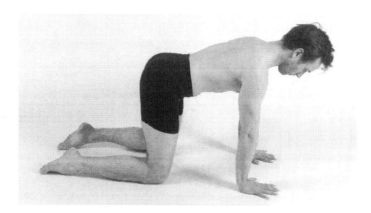

Kneeling and Standing

Next, reach your arms towards the ceiling, continuing to keep your abs held strong while breathing in and out effortlessly.

Lastly, while standing, reach your arms towards the ceiling, continuing to keep your abs held strong while breathing in and out effortlessly.

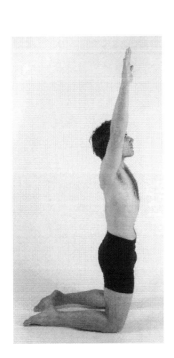
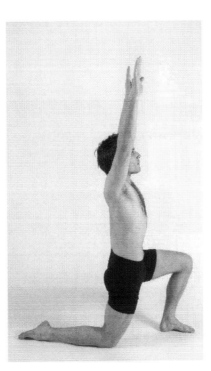
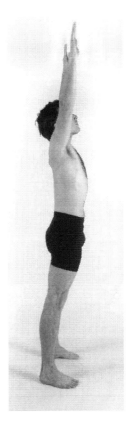

 VIDEO 2: KNEELING TO STANDING ABDOMINAL BRACING

The Truth about Stretching

It's hazardous not to stretch. However, there are limitations to what stretching can do for you. It's a fallacy to believe that if you stretch your muscles they will remain lengthened. The fact is, if you cannot touch your toes today, and you stretch tonight and achieve the ability to touch your toes, when you wake up tomorrow, the likelihood is that you probably will be short and tight again, and thus, unable to touch your toes. That's because you are only as flexible as your anatomy will allow. If you were flexible as a child, then you could retain this flexibility. However, if you were never really flexible, you probably will never be flexible. Stretching is meant to relax muscles and create a state of being limber. It breaks down unwanted scar tissue adhesions from acts of exercise or inflammation from tension over strain or injury. The problem is that people with low back pain generally stretch the wrong way, stretch the wrong muscles, or stretch at the wrong time of day. I'm here to make sense of it all for you.

Twenty years ago, research about muscle stretching started and was instantly divided into two camps—half of the experts believed that stretching was good for you while the other half determined it was bad. Well, guess what—both camps are right. The truth is that stretching is good for you but it's not great if you just target your spinal muscles, especially if you've hurt your back. You need to stretch the muscles that affect the back, as opposed to directly stretching the spine.

Here are some facts:

1. Stretching prior to physical activity is associated with a 33% greater risk of injury and a 33% decrease in strength. This means you can injure your muscles with only two thirds of the force you might otherwise need. With this information in mind, why would you even think of stretching your injured back before taking a walk or moving from the couch to your desk?

2. Muscles already shorten and lengthen repeatedly during any activity and seldom achieve the range of motion demanded by most flexibility routines. When you perform a stretch and hold it, you create a neuro-muscular response, or adaptation. That is, you're teaching your brain to tolerate the strain associated with stretching, leaving the muscles less responsive and weakened. This is why stretching your back is not a great way to wake up your body and prepare it for movement. Stretching is a much better way to end your day by doing a series of safe and effective stretches before you go to sleep.

3. If you've injured your back, you've likely caused some degree of tearing or displacement to a muscle, ligament, or joint. Why would you stretch an already injured muscle when this will just make it even weaker and less responsive? Please understand, I am not telling you not to stretch, I am telling you not to stretch your back muscles directly. There are better ways to limber up your spine without actually directing all flexibility to the muscles which are achy, sore, or inflamed. First, we need to figure out how to limber up without causing further harm to your spine.

How to Limber Up Your Low Back without Stretching

I've seen patients endlessly stretch stiff and sore joints. As I said, injury causes ripping and tearing to the connective tissues that hold your spine together. By stretching these tissues, you are provoking further injury and promoting instability.

When you first injure your back, the stiffening is protecting against further injury. Most people want to stretch out their spine because it feels so stiff. This is backwards thinking. For example, did you know that most back attacks occur after stretching stiff backs in the morning, often by trying to bend forward and touch your toes as soon as you climb out of bed?

During sleep, the spine draws fluid into the discs between your vertebrae, promoting hydration. This is an important physiological process called "imbibition". It nourishes the gel within the disks to keep them hydrated. This drawing in of fluid actually makes you taller in the morning. All those discs are full of nourishing, hydrating fluid and they increase the space between vertebrae, lengthening your spine.

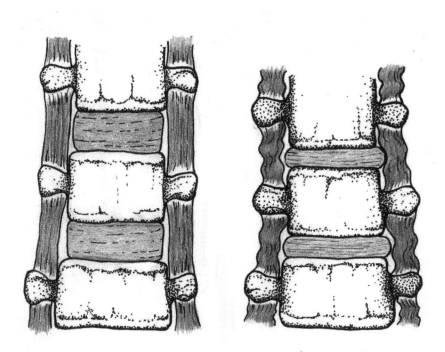

Diagram 4: Morning disc swelling (left) and evening disc compression (right)

While imbibition is an important physiological method of nourishing the discs, the larger size means the spinal ligaments attaching one vertebra to another are like an overstretched rubber band, providing less support. This is why, if you bend forward and touch your toes, stoop, slouch, or pull your knees to your chest, especially in the morning, you run the risk of injury and can buckle your back.

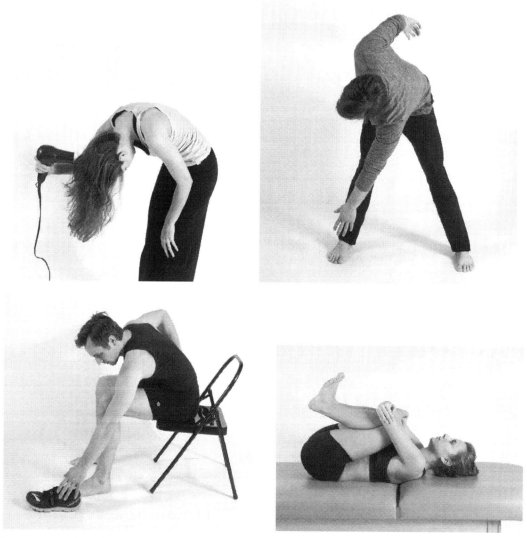

Movements that risk injury and can buckle your spine when performed in the morning

Awaken Your Spine

I have created *Back in Action* spinal exercises that promote movement without stretching and without the associated risk of injury. Think of these exercises as preparing your body for motion. They are safe exercises that lubricate the joints, reduce inflammation, wake up muscles and tendons, and activate and protect your spine. They also encourage normal biomechanics and prevent the unwanted buildup of scar tissue adhesions. Scar tissue is a byproduct of inflammation and injury. It can aggregate and form nodules and knots, which stick to adjacent soft tissue structures. These knots alter how tissues glide over each other, resulting in abnormal movement and limited range of motion, or locking up of your spine.

Ever get a massage? It feels great, but the effects are not long lasting if you don't incorporate movement into your routine following the massage. In fact, your condition may even worsen because the scar tissue might not have been completely broken down and can reform because of inflammation caused by the compression of the massage. You can prevent this by continuing to move and loosen the unwanted adhesions within your muscles and spinal joints.

This is where your participation is essential. Develop a daily habit for taking care of your lower back. You know enough now to know what's good and what's bad for your spine. Follow my guidelines and by the end of a few weeks, you will be "Back in Action."

3

YOUR BACK IN ACTION ROUTINE

*"The art of medicine consists of amusing the
patient while Nature cures the disease."*

—VOLTAIRE

THINK ABOUT SOMEONE WHO has a serious knee injury. When a surgeon
repairs or replaces a knee joint, the "hardware" has changed, but what about
the "software"? Before the operation, the person with the bum knee had likely
been walking around on a bad limb for many years before finally making the
decision to repair it. The common compensation is to avoid putting weight on
that leg. The entire body adapts to this abnormal movement pattern, which,
by now, probably feels normal. Now, all of a sudden, the knee is new but old
habits die hard. Traditional rehabilitation models use weights to strengthen
those joints and retrain the brain to go along with new movements.

This strategy doesn't work with the spine. Simply strengthening the spine after an injury and years of abnormal movement patterns will lock your back into an abnormal posture. First, you have to restore motion to the spinal joints. Then, limber up the muscles which tug and shear against the spine. Finally, the back must be strengthened. Unfortunately, this is hardly ever done or done in the correct sequence. Most patients, when I first meet them, tell me of past back attacks which were treated by strength exercises. Essentially, the back was hurt and then locked into that abnormal posture by some unwitting doctor or therapist. Complete mayhem ensued!

At this point, I want to teach you how to train your core/torso muscles to kick in quickly and protect your spine from unguarded movements, slips, and falls. We need to break old habits and replace them with a new set of instructions. There's no magic bullet; no one special exercise that will rid you of your back pain. Instead, there are special action sequences which strengthen your spine and protect your back. I've developed a routine to safely protect your back. They are meant to help overwrite your old software and protect your hardware—your spine.

So, read on. You're almost there. Remember, this is a journey with a destination of permanent relief of low back pain, and the steps are clearly laid out for you right here.

The *Back in Action* Program

Perform the *Back in Action* exercises listed below to safely limber up your spine and reduce pain. These movements lessen the load and loosen and activate the muscles needed to support your posture without the risks associated with stretching. Just ten seconds for each movement is adequate to get the benefits from them. In this case, more is actually better. Try them all to begin with. If one or more particular movements feel really good, enjoy the motion and stay with it a little longer. There's no set formula; perform as many or as few exercises as you want, but make sure to perform them smoothly. Remember that these are not stretches, so keep moving back and forth through the exercises. Take your time now to heal faster. This is where your participation is essential. Develop a habit for taking care of your lower back. You're prepared enough now to know what's good and what's bad for your spine.

Back in Action Routines

Morning Stiffness: Dynamically wake up your postural muscles while lubricating your joints so you can start your day pain free.

Workday Tension: "Back breaks" help maintain low back mobility while in an office setting.

Evening Decompression: Floor movements to relieve low back compression.

Daily Stretches: Five essential stretches which save your spine from arthritis.

Core Stability: Endurance exercises which build a corset of strength to protect your back.

Abdominal Bracing: Quickly engages your abs & teaches your nervous system to protect your spine. (Daily Habit)

Baby Steps

I believe in taking small steps to achieve success with my low back program. I recommend the 4-week plan: it adds one element of the *Back in Action* movement program each week to help resolve lower back pain.

Once you complete the 4-week plan, tie it all together by using the protocols outlined in the *Back in Action* program.

Have fun with the movements—identify the ones which help you the most and create a routine that helps resolve your low back pain. Think of this program as an exercise diet: there's not one way to use the program, but many ways to incorporate it into your life. Once you figure out which stretches, movements and core endurance exercises help you the most, fit them into your lifestyle. Next is a synopsis for the entire *Back in Action* program with suggested frequency.

Morning Stiffness Routines

We already know that sleeping hydrates your disks, making them vulnerable to injury. My recommended movement routine helps redistribute and lessen the intervertebral disc pressure, essentially taking the load off your back via imbibition—the transfer of fluids from one solid to the next, aided by motion. Do this movement routine when you wake up in the morning and are stiff. It moves the fluid around and takes pressure off the discs and lubricates the joints. Once motion is begun, the spinal joints start lubricating themselves and redistributing stagnant synovial fluid, which has been stuck within the joint due to immobility. Synovial fluid is your body's natural oil; once redistributed, it creates an effect of limbering stiff joints. These movements not only help the joints, but also assist sore muscles by waking up specific postural muscles that have been inactive. The movement routine is broken down into two sections: a standing routine and a floor routine.

I created these routines to wake up your muscles, lubricate your joints, and activate your body so that it's ready for the demands of your day. I suggest you try all of them for ten seconds each and then pick and choose the ones that make your back feel the best. Once you've arrived at your optimal personalized routine and you're feeling really good, you can do them for as long as you want. They work as both treatments of back pain and as a preventative measure.

Morning Stiffness Standing Routine

Time commitment: 2 minutes

Sky Reaches

Keeping your torso straight, extend each hand and bend slightly to the side with an emphasis on lifting your rib cage and breathing in as you reach upwards on both sides. You should feel a release of flanks and the ability to take a deep breath.

Benefits: Lubricates the joints of the upper back and acts as a beginning pattern of movement that lifts the ribs and decompresses the spine.

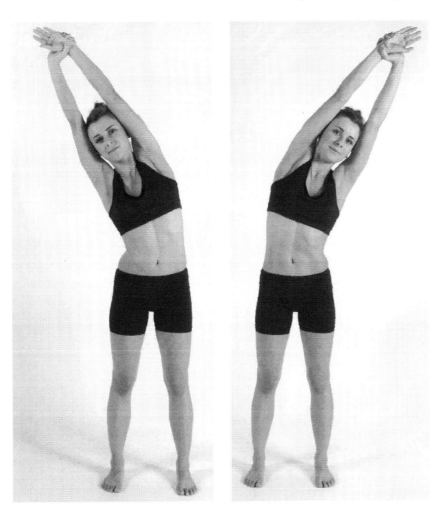

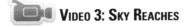 **VIDEO 3: SKY REACHES**

Swimmer

Extend arms and move in a forward, circular, motion—line swimming the freestyle stroke. You should rotate your mid-back as you swing your arms. You may feel a release from the front of your shoulders and upper torso.

Benefits: Multi-joint action of the shoulder blade over the mid torso, involving a gentle rotary movement to the rib cage, which is a very stiff area in the mid-part of the spine.

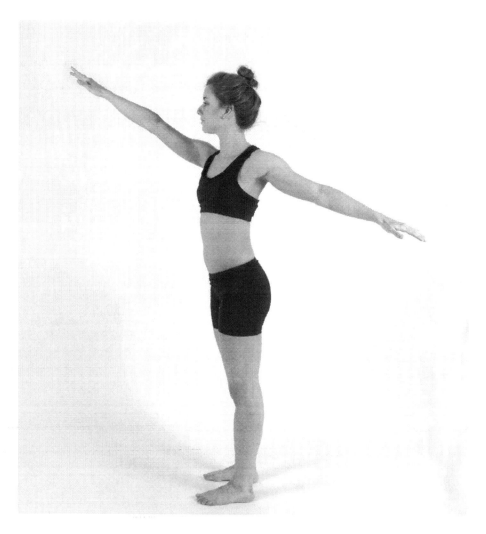

VIDEO 4: SWIMMER

Backstroke

Extend arms like in swimmer and rotate them backwards in a circular motion as if you're swimming the backstroke. Allow your upper body to rotate. You should feel a release in the back of your shoulders and your middle torso.

Benefits: Targets the spinal erectors and muscles beneath the shoulder blades that are essential to preventing a rounded upper back posture.

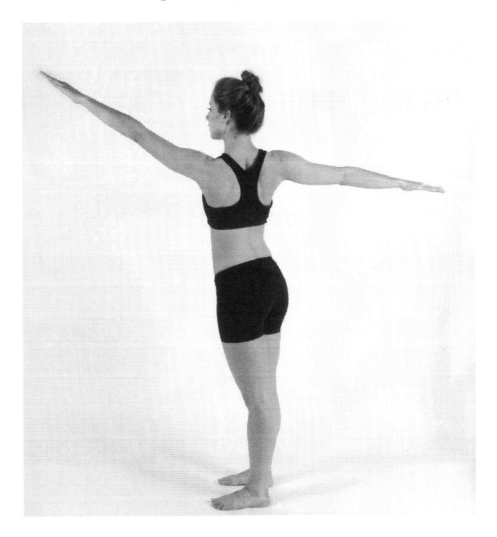

VIDEO 5: BACKSTROKE

Standing Angel

To do this easy, three-part move. First, bring your hands up and together so that the palms are toward your face, raising them together above your head. Next, part them by squeezing your shoulder blades together. Then, slowly lower your elbows toward your back pockets. Then start again. You should feel a release of tension in your shoulder blades and the bottom of your neck.

Benefits: I call this a perfect posture movement, which helps prevent the rounded shoulder appearance by helping to glide the shoulder blades back onto the thoracic wall.

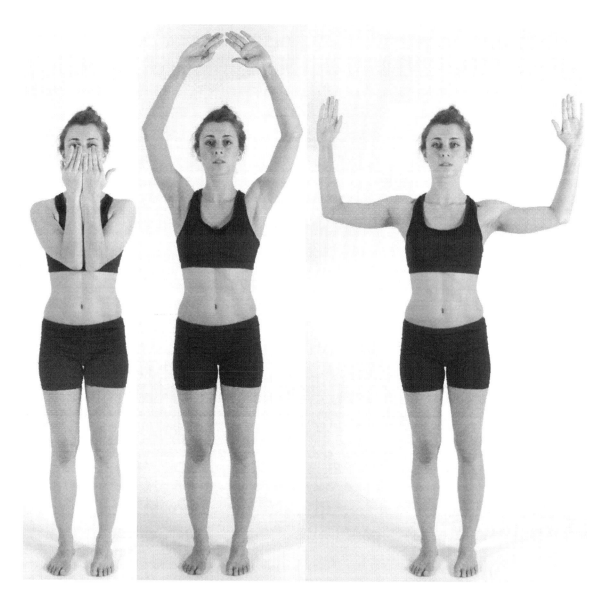

📹 VIDEO 6: ANGELS

Golf Twists

With your feet shoulder-width apart, fold your arms across your chest, keeping your head facing forward, and twist your body from side to side.

Benefits: Lubricates joints between the rib cage and lower back, creating a separation of the lower back, loosening the spinal facet joints while sending excitatory messages to the spinal erector muscles to "wake up" the multifidi, the muscles responsible for rotating the spine. These muscles have been connected to atrophy and complaints of chronic low back pain.

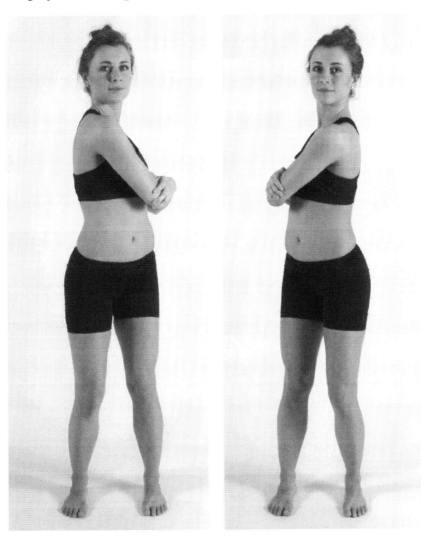

VIDEO 7: GOLF TWISTS

Pelvic Twist

Cross arms in front of you at shoulder level and twist from left to right with your pelvis, moving the bottom half of your torso and legs with each twist, with an emphasis on keeping your upper body still. You should feel like Chuck Berry doing the twist. Furthermore, you may hear and feel a release from the upper portion of your lower back.

Benefits: The release from the upper portion of your lower back creates a sense of mobility and separation/proprioception awareness. Joints between the lower back and pelvis are also lubricated with this motion.

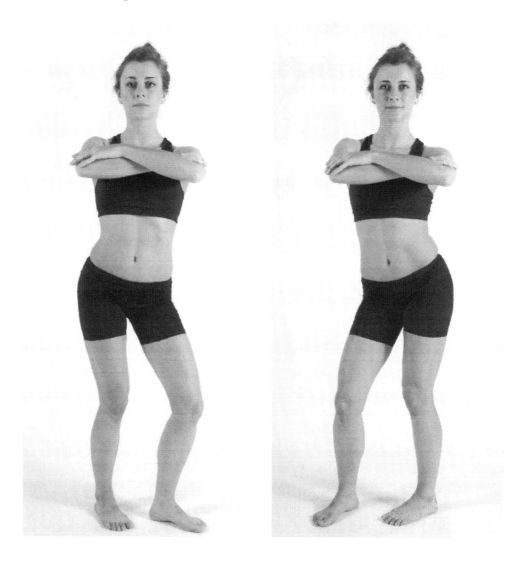

VIDEO 8: PELVIC TWIST

Pelvic Thrust

Standing still, sway your lower back and then flatten it. You should feel a release of tension from the lower back. With your feet shoulder-width apart, fold your arms across your chest, tuck your belly button in toward your spine, and tuck in your pelvis. Then, reverse the motion by arching your back. This anterior-to-posterior gliding movement exaggerates a swayback posture and then transitions to a pelvic tuck or flat back.

Benefits: Essential movement that lubricates lower back joints. It targets the pelvic deep muscles to provide a communicative link between the lower back, pelvis, and lower extremities.

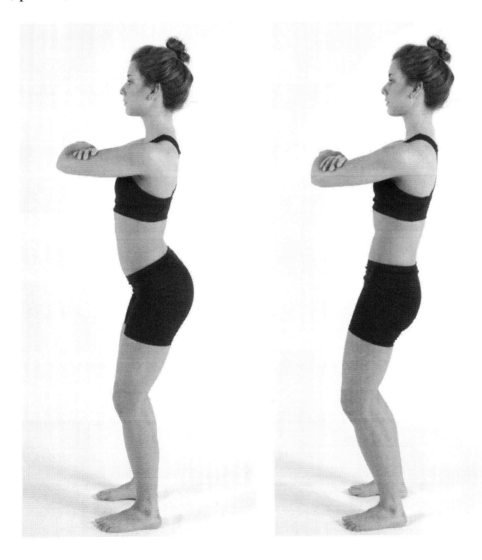

VIDEO 10: PELVIC THRUST

Pelvic Clocks

Standing with feet shoulder-width apart, slowly move your hips and pelvis as if you were playing with a hula hoop, slowly gyrating your belly button in a circular pattern. Think of Hawaiian dances at a luau.

Benefits: This oscillating movement pattern provides a communicative link between the lumbar spine, pelvis, and lower extremities, and it is very soothing for the lower back.

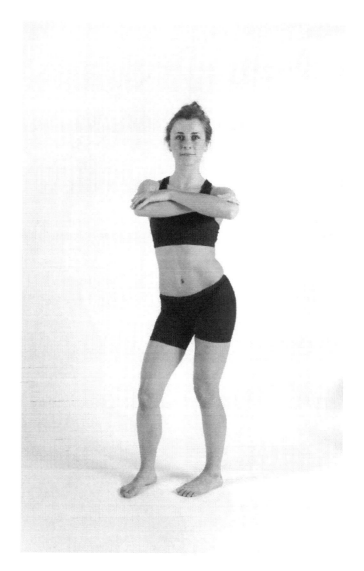

VIDEO 9: PELVIC CLOCKS

Hip Gyro

The hips are ball-and-socket joints. The emphasis of this motion is to move the hip in an outward circular motion. You should feel a release of tension from the hip sockets and groin.

Benefits: Activates the internal and external rotators of the hip while creating a comfortable range of motion in the socket. It also lubricates the hip joint and helps to prevent arthritic change from a lack of mobility. The hip is meant to perform a semi-circular movement, but very rarely do we ever achieve this motion, as we simply move forward or backward in most situations.

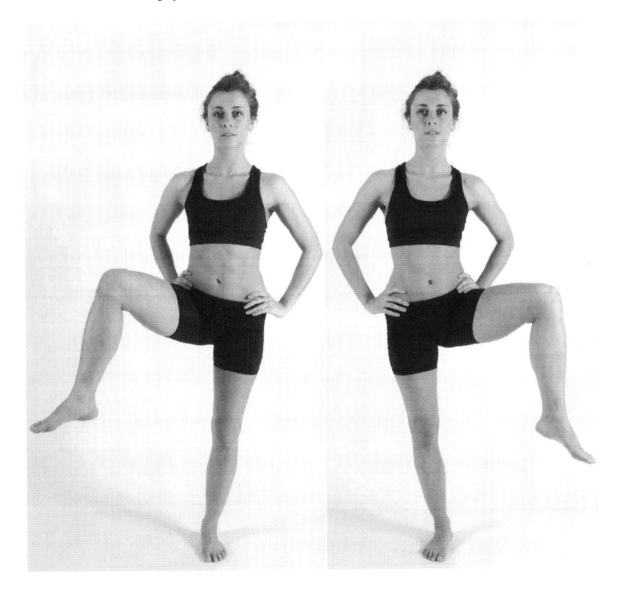

VIDEO **11**: HIP GYRO

Leg Swings

By performing leg swings you activate the core abdominal muscles, spinal erectors, hip flexors, and hip extensors all at once. Simply stand on one leg, hold your balance or hold onto a wall or counter top, and gently swing your leg straight out in front and then behind you.

Benefits: Dynamically wakes up the both the front and rear of the thighs, helping create an improved range of motion in a forward plane. It lubricates the hip socket with synovial fluid and helps break down adhesions which limit mobility in the hip flexors and hip extensors (preventing cartilage tears, muscle pulls, and strains).

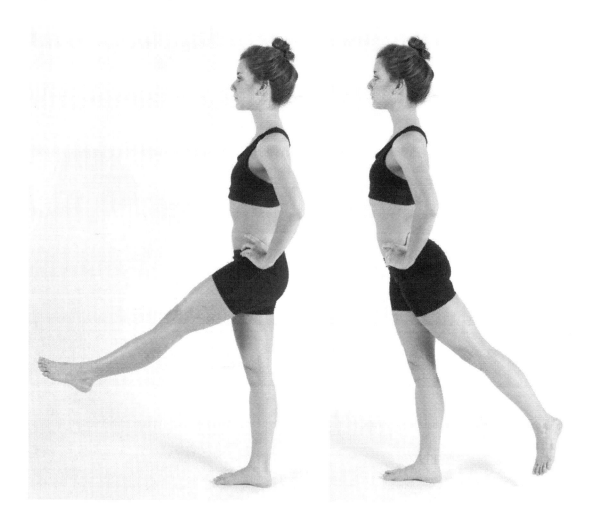

VIDEO 16: LEG SWINGS

Diagonal Leg Swing

Diagonal leg swings are performed like regular leg swings but on an angle, which helps break up scar tissue adhesions that form in the inner thigh and groin.

Benefits: Similar to leg swings but adding motion to the inner thigh. This motion simultaneously breaks down unwanted joint adhesions while stretching and activating the entire hip socket. Hence, getting you ready to ambulate.

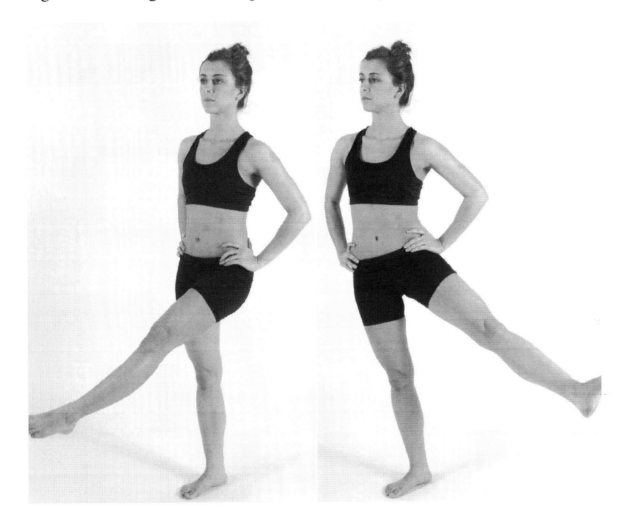

VIDEO 17: DIAGONAL LEG SWINGS

Lunge and Reach

Lunge forward, first with the right and then with the left leg. As you lunge, reach up to the sky with the opposite arm and bend to the side. The emphasis is on lifting the rib cage toward the ceiling. Reverse the position. You should feel a release of tension through the upper thigh and rib cage.

Benefits: Wakes up the glutes, especially the gluteus medius, which helps keep a level pelvis. It also prevents hip drop posture while simultaneously stretching out the front of the thigh and hips, creating elasticity to the hip flexors while co-activating the hip extensors. Furthermore, it creates a rib cage lift that helps with releasing diaphragmatic adhesions and eases breathing while mimicking spinal decompression. It's what we ask of our body and rarely achieve. This is a personal favorite and go-to exercise of mine.

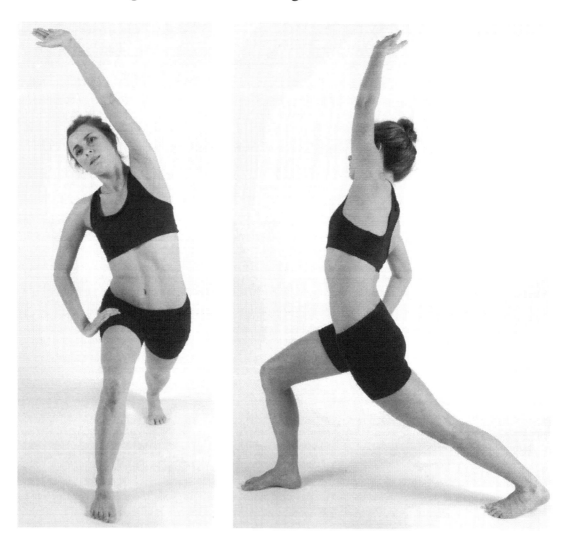

📹 VIDEO 12: LUNGE AND REACH

Bowling

Stand with your legs apart and slide one leg diagonally behind you (as in a release in bowling) while supporting your body with your opposite hip. Hold your arms out for balance and repeat on the other side. You should feel tension build in your supportive leg and outer buttocks.

Benefits: This movement will wake up your gluteus medius, the muscle that helps keep your pelvis equally balanced when you stand, walk, and run.

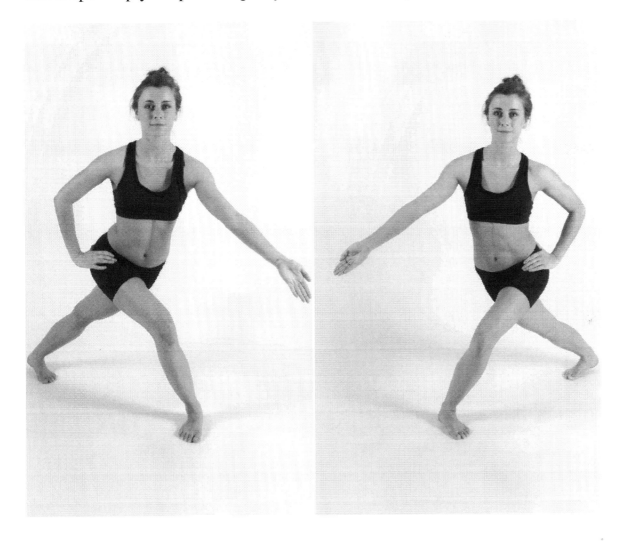

VIDEO **13**: BOWLING

Hacky Sack

While maintaining your balance, lift your leg up, flex your knee out, and try to touch your hand to your ankle. Hold on to a railing with the opposite arm if necessary. You should feel a release of tension of the sciatic muscle or outer buttocks.

Benefits: It targets the sciatic notch in prevention of sciatic nerve pain. It is also a movement that limbers the piriformis muscle, which adheres or surrounds the area around the sciatic nerve, preventing adhesions from forming around the nerve. It works on balance and preparedness to maintain balance, while simultaneously limbering and waking up the back part of the hips.

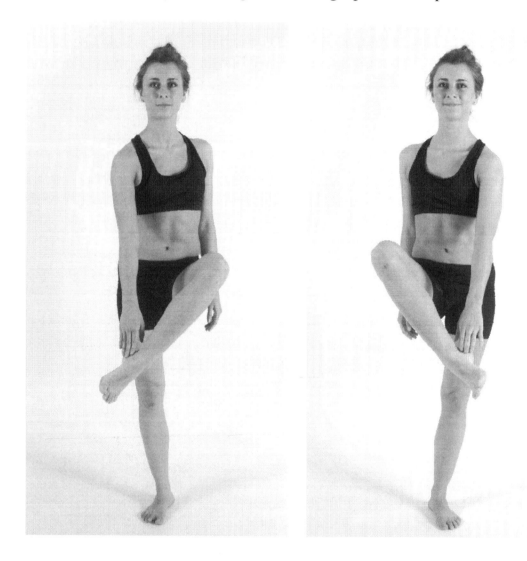

VIDEO 14: HACKY SACK

Counter Traction*

Find a stable counter top that is about waist-high and support your upper body while allowing your legs to dangle. You should feel a release of pressure from your middle to lower back. While ensuring a stable surface that can support your body weight, simply use your upper-body arm strength to lift yourself so that your toes are just about to leave the ground. It's a convenient way to use your body as leverage and create spinal decompression. Avoid if you have shoulder problems or if you lack upper body strength.

Benefits: A creative way to use your body weight to provide spinal traction and decompression.

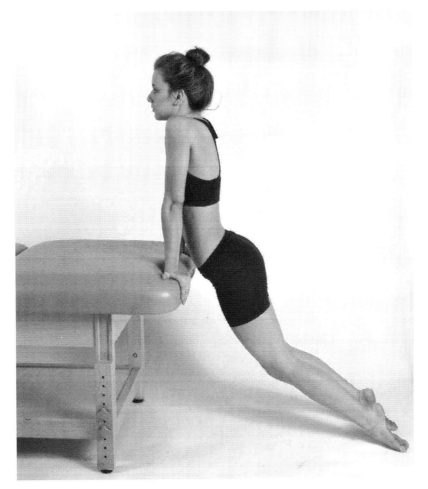

*AVOID THIS EXERCISE IF YOU HAVE A SHOULDER INJURY.

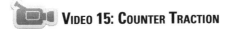 VIDEO 15: COUNTER TRACTION

Morning Stiffness Floor Routine

Time commitment: 3 minutes

Descending Hip Drops

On your back, lift your legs in the air as if you're sitting in a chair. Keeping arms out to the side for balance, drop your hips from side to side. Perform this action until the feet are against the floor.

Benefits: This is a great way to provide movement for the lower spine. It literally targets the entire mid and lower back. While the focus is to slowly drop your hips from side to side, this motion introduces mobility to the spinal joints and helps break up unwanted adhesions that may possibly lock your facet joints and limit your mobility. It's not unusual to feel a pop or a click that releases CO_2 gas and promotes spinal mobility.

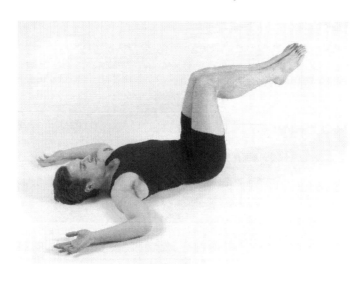

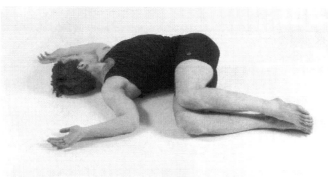

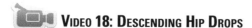 **VIDEO 18: DESCENDING HIP DROPS**

Pelvic Release

Lie on your back, cross one ankle on top of the opposite knee, and slowly pull that knee to the floor with your ankle. This will provide a slow stretching motion to the outer thigh, known as your IT band. The movement stops when the opposing knee is almost touching the floor.

Benefits: This movement is designed to gently release the sacroiliac joint of the pelvis, which is often associated with low back pain. This is a challenging area due to spinal stiffness and adhesions to the iliotibial band, commonly known as the IT band. The IT band runs from the outer thigh to the knee. Because of its biomechanical attachments to both the pelvis and the knees, the IT band tugs on the knee cap and pulls it out of alignment when overactive. Now not only do you have low back pain but knee pain as well. The pelvic release is also a great movement and prep exercise to mobilize your spine. Don't be surprised if you hear a pop or a click; it's probably adhesions being released from the spine as a result of this added mobility. Consider this a kinetic chain approach to solving lower back pain. This is another one of my go-to exercises for spinal mobility and relief of unwanted spinal pressure. I simply love this movement.

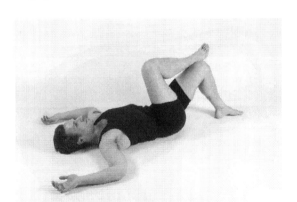 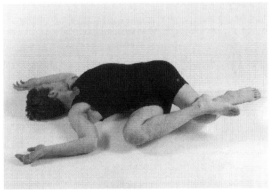

VIDEO 19: PELVIC RELEASE

Back Bridges

Lie on your back, tighten your abdominal muscles, lift your butt from the floor, and keep your torso in line with your thighs. You will feel a tightening in the back of your thighs and glutes, as well as the abdominals. This is called co-activation and is essential to spine stabilization because the simultaneous working of the back and front parts of your midsection will create a corset of strength around your lower back.

Benefits: This exercise creates a neuromuscular activation to teach your body to co-activate both the abdominal wall and your spinal erectors at the same time, which is an essential process for lower back stabilization.

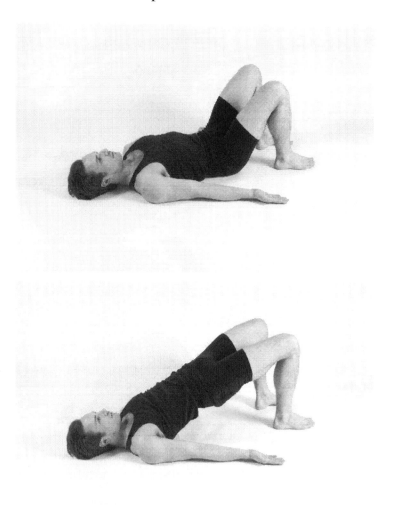

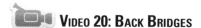 VIDEO 20: BACK BRIDGES

Marching Bridge

Same as back bridge, but now march in place.

Benefits: Same as Back Bridges; however, this movement challenges the core and spinal erectors and fires the glute muscles to help prevent a hip-drop posture while standing, walking, or running.

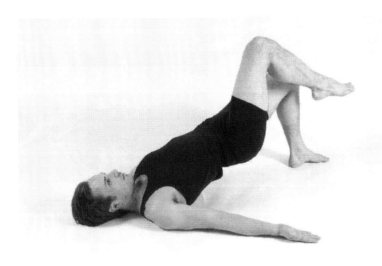

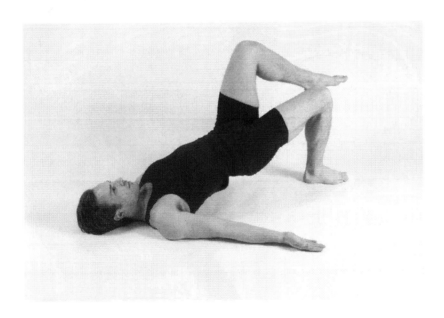

VIDEO 21: MARCHING BRIDGE

Knee Hugs Bridge

Same as Back Bridges, but now pull one knee towards your chest as you balance on the other leg.

Benefits: The most challenging of all the bridge routines, this will demand your core, spinal erectors, and glutes to support your back while you activate and engage your hips, essentially getting you ready to walk, stand, or run. It also releases tension and adhesions from the hip/groin that mimic a pinched feeling in the hip socket.

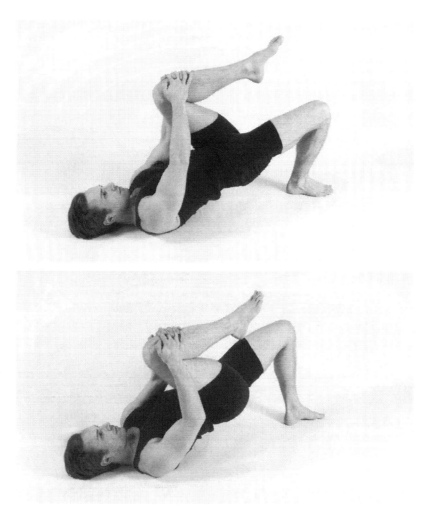

VIDEO 22: KNEE HUGS BRIDGE

Dynamic Hamstrings

On your back, with your knees bent and feet on the floor, grab your right thigh with both hands, then straighten and bend your knee back and forth. Repeat with the left thigh.

Benefits: This exercise lubricates the knee joints by engaging your hamstrings and creates an active range of motion of the hips and pelvis by providing a nice blood supply to the hamstrings to keep them active and moist. This movement contrasts with a stretch-and-hold posture that deactivates the hamstring; not what you need when you are trying to start your day.

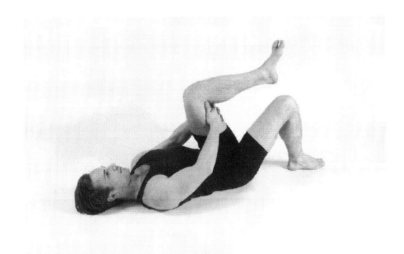

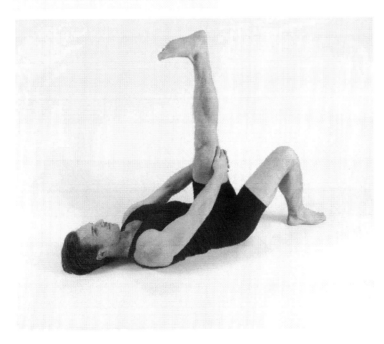

VIDEO 23: DYNAMIC HAMSTRING

Hip Openers*

Lie on your back, and bend both of your knees while keeping your feet on the floor. Cross one ankle over the other knee and gently push and pull the knee of the crossed ankle in and out.

Benefits: This exercise works to open the hip sockets, maintaining motion within the joint space while breaking down unwanted adhesions that limit mobility. It also helps to prevent cartilage and labral tears in the hip socket.

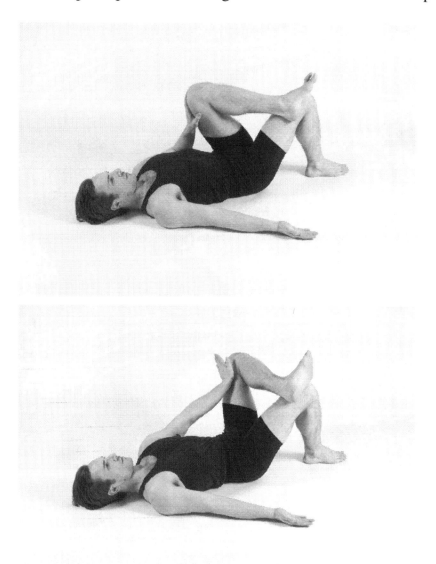

*AVOID THIS EXERCISE IF YOU HAVE HAD A HIP REPLACEMENT.

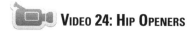 VIDEO 24: HIP OPENERS

Windshield Wipers

Lie on your back, bend your knees, and lift your ankles from the floor as if you were in a seated posture while lying on your back. Then, place your fists together between your knees and squeeze your knees together, putting pressure on your fists. Turn your ankles in and out, rotating your shins like a windshield wiper.

Benefits: This exercise uses a small but critical range of movement for the hip socket and activates your internal rotators, allowing for complete lubrication of the ball and socket joint. The importance of these muscles and joints should never be overlooked.

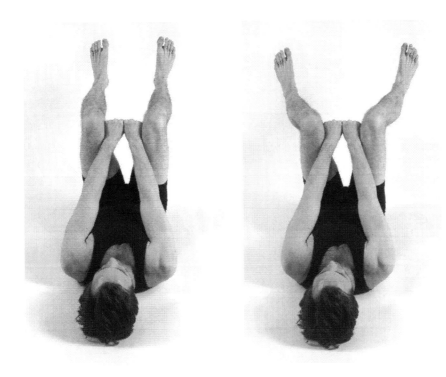

VIDEO 25: WINDSHIELD WIPERS

Clam Shell

Lie on your side in a fetal position and stack your ankles on top of each other. Keeping your feet together, open your knees as much as possible.

Benefits: This is an elementary exercise that targets the external rotators of the hip to ensure a level pelvis while upright. It's a very easy and effective way to prepare your hips for maintaining your body weight and not placing the entire load on your spine. It also wakes up your outer hips.

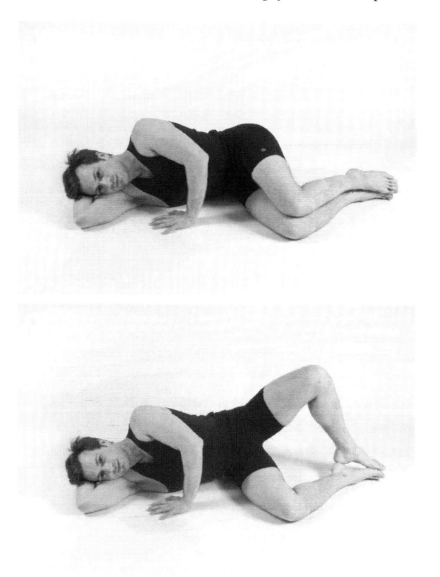

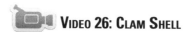 VIDEO 26: CLAM SHELL

Dynamic Hip Flexors

Lie down on your side and pull your bottom leg up toward your chest. Use your top arm to grab your top foot or knee (hold wherever is most comfortable for you). Flex your knee and thigh to your chest, then try to pull your heel to your buttock.

Benefits: This action lubricates your hip sockets and wakes up both your hip flexors and hip extensors while lubricating and preventing hip impingement, or that pinching feeling in the groin when adhesions are formed. This movement is essential in preventing sway-back postures.

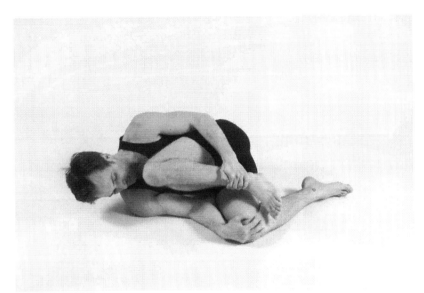

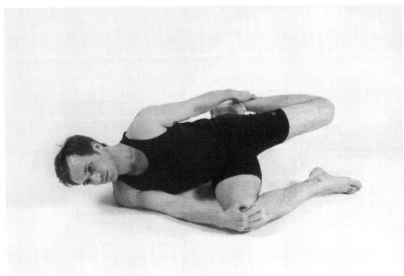

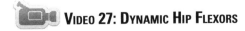 **VIDEO 27: DYNAMIC HIP FLEXORS**

Open Book

Lie on your side in a fetal position with your arms straight out in front of you. Open up your body like you would a book, making sure to keep your legs together on the floor while twisting your torso.

Benefits: This exercise is another of my favorites. It enhances your body's ability to provide much-needed motion to the transition area of the spine, where the highly rigid rib cage meets the highly moveable lower back. This is a common area of arthritic change in most individuals.

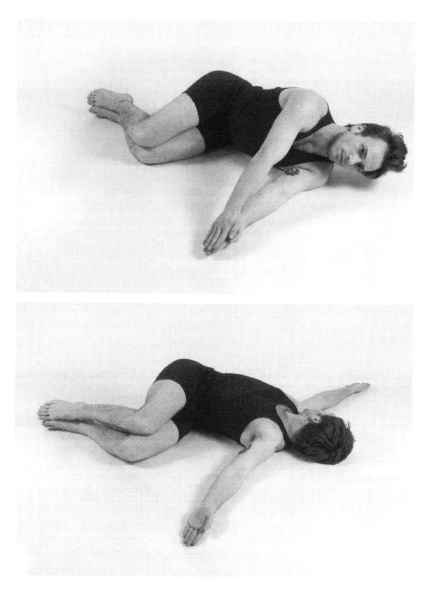

VIDEO 28: OPEN BOOK

Ab Curls

Lying on your back, flex one knee and keep your foot flat on the floor while the other leg remains stretched out. This ensures a level pelvis and a relaxed hip flexor mechanism. Then, place your hands palms down under your buttocks and perform an abdominal curl just to the point where your shoulder blades are off the floor. Hold for 5 seconds and repeat on the other side.

Benefits: Building your core is essential to preventing lower back pain and this movement does exactly that. It wakes up the abdominal wall while taking out the havoc that the hip flexors may cause from the shearing effect on the spine.

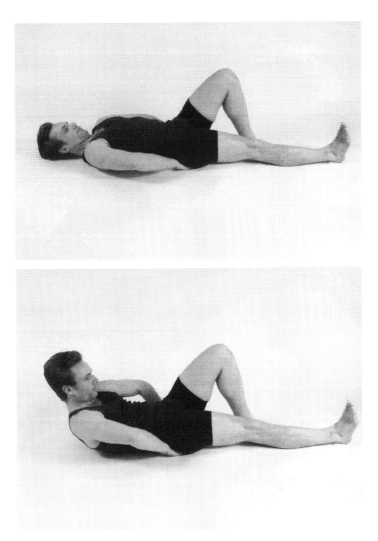

VIDEO 29: AB CURLS

Front Plank

Start in a push-up position, only balancing your weight on your forearms. Make sure that your elbows are flexed instead of placing all your weight on your wrists.

Benefits: This is a core activity that wakes up the transversus abdominus and helps transfer energy of movement from the upper body to the lower body without placing the strain of the load on your spine.

Alternate Method: If it is too challenging, place a cushion under your knees caps and balance from that posture. Just cross your ankle and lift from the floor.

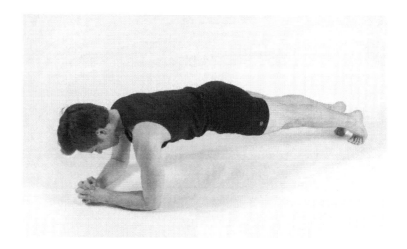

VIDEO 30: FRONT PLANK

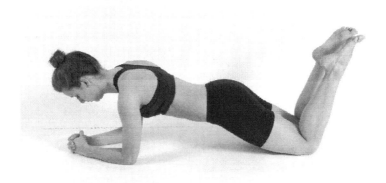

VIDEO 63: HALF PLANK

Side Bridges

Next, from a plank position, try to roll to your side, balancing on your forearm and ankles only. Elevate everything else from the floor. Then, try to keep your torso stiff and roll to the other side.

Benefits: The benefits are similar to those of the front plank, only the side plank is more challenging and involves the abdominal obliques and the diagonal muscles that wrap around your pelvis. This action helps to create a full abdominal corset of stability and forms a hoop of strength to protect your spine.

Alternate Method: If it is too challenging, lay on your side, shoulder on ground stacked on top of each other and simply lift your legs upward towards the ceiling keeping ankles stacked on top of each other.

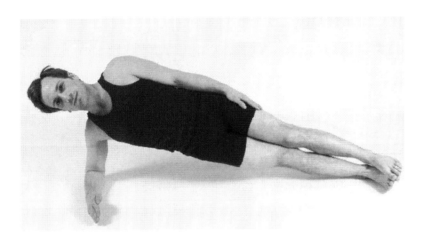

VIDEO 31: SIDE BRIDGES

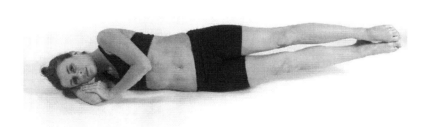

VIDEO 68: STRAIGHT-LEG TORSO LIFT

Reach-Backs

On all fours, place one hand behind your head and reach down, touching your elbow to the inside of the straight arm. Then, reach in the opposite direction by pointing your elbow toward the ceiling and let your gaze follow your moving arm.

Benefits: This movement lubricates your middle back and shoulders and creates mobility in the stiff transitional zone of the spine between your mid-back/rib cage and your lower back. At the same time, this exercise wakes up the spinal rotators, which are generally atrophied and weak in people who suffer from chronic back pain.

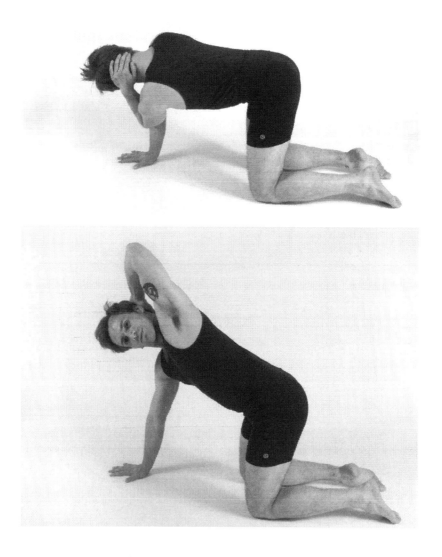

VIDEO 32: REACH-BACKS

Point and Reach

On all fours, balance on your hands and knees. Reach forward with one arm, keeping your balance, and then stretch out the opposite leg. The goal here is to reach as far forward and as far back as possible with the opposite arm and leg while also keeping your balance and abdominal brace. This will create co-activation of both the front and back of the core at the same time. Touch your elbow to your knee and repeat, then switch sides.

Benefits: This exercise activates the spinal erectors and hip extensors with minimal loading and prepares them to hold your spine upright.

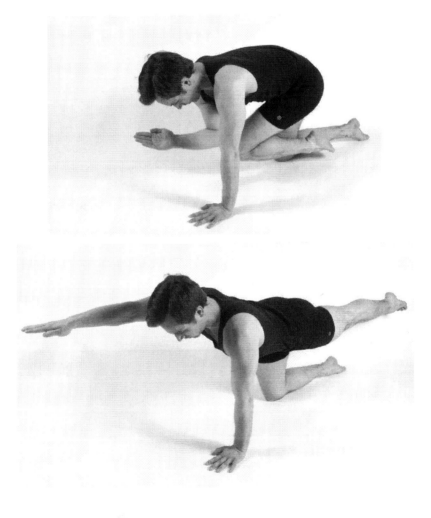

VIDEO 33: POINT AND REACH

Cat and Cow

On all fours, round your back and drop your head forward. Reverse this action by arching your back and extending your head up, looking at the ceiling. Focus on flaring and pinching your shoulder blades as you move.

Benefits: This movement provides full spinal lubrication which readies the spine for movement, enhancing both flexion and extension in a safe, effective way.

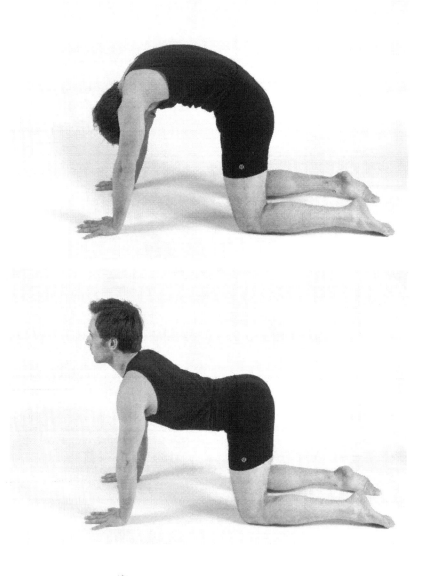

📹 VIDEO 34: CAT AND COW

Abdominal Brace on all Fours

While on your hands and knees, arch and sway your lower back until you find a comfortable and neutral low back posture, then tighten the abdominals to hold that posture and stand up. Imagine someone is about to punch you in the stomach and tighten all your abs in an instant.

Benefits: Learning to engage your core is essential for spinal stability. Ending with this movement ensures you stabilize what you just accomplished with the previous stretches and exercises—a great way to end the routine and lock in the benefits.

For now, try learning the basics. The next time you're seated, try the following routine: Tighten your buttocks and focus on the sensation of touching the seat. Next, tighten and relax different muscles in your body, such as your arms, thighs, calves, neck, etc. Now, feel your abs and try to tighten and relax them. Look in the mirror if you need visual feedback. Lastly, try bracing; tighten your buttocks and abs at the same time while making sure you don't hold your breath.

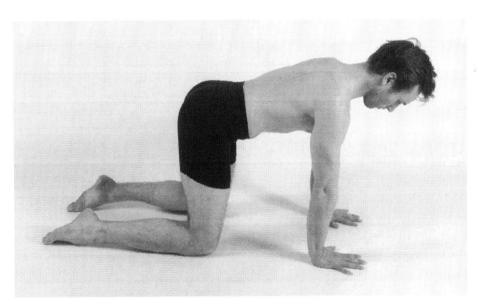

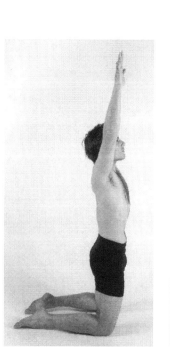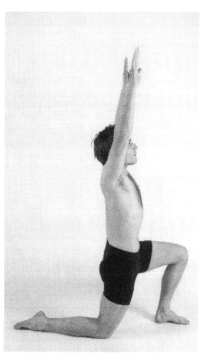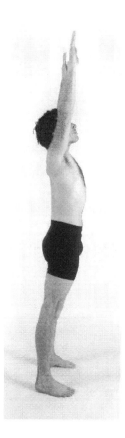

VIDEO 2: KNEELING TO STANDING ABDOMINAL BRACING

Congratulations! You are ready to start your day.

Workday Tension Routines

It's essential to get some back movements in during your workday—especially if you are at a job where you sit at a desk all day, travel long distances on planes, or following your daily commute have to sit at a desk for extended periods. The program below is essential to prevent low back pain. Being seated is what really creates havoc on the lower back, as it loses its natural curve and begins to flatten. This places pressure on the discs and can make them bulge or protrude backward towards the spinal canal where there are painful nerve endings and joints. The ligaments of the back, which are supposed to be short and supportive, begin to stretch out and lose their integrity, calling muscles into play that aren't trained to handle the endurance necessary for this activity. This scenario creates an environment of spinal instability in which your back can buckle or a disk can herniate. It can also exacerbate an already painful spine condition.

These at-work exercises take only a few minutes of your time—less than a coffee break. You'll still have time to go to the kitchen and make some tea or take a stroll to the water cooler.

Perform the following seated movement routine as a complete set throughout your working day to help normalize your posture and relieve stress in your spine. It only takes about 90 seconds. Furthermore, you can perform it as many times as necessary to make you feel comfortable. You can't overdo the frequency of these work-related movements.

Workday Tension Seated Routine

Time commitment: 90 seconds

Seated Sky Reaches

These are the same as Standing Reaches, but performed in the seated position. Reach upward and across your body while alternating arms and breathing in deeply.

Benefits: This movement promotes an upright posture while creating spinal decompression from the facet joints and discs.

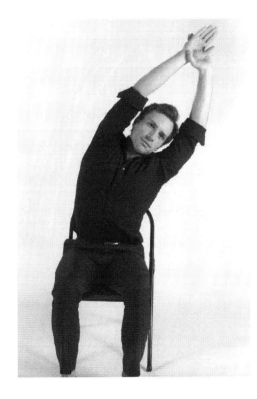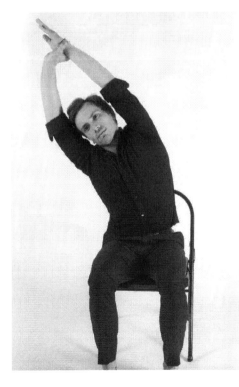

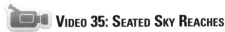 **VIDEO 35: SEATED SKY REACHES**

Seated Angels

Sit up straight and lift your arms above your head, pressing your hands together. Next, bring your arms down to your sides, pressing your arms back with palms forward. Then repeat. You should feel tension build in your middle back and release in your shoulders.

Benefits: This stretch wakes up the mid-back muscles that deactivate when you are in a seated position. It also prevents a rounded shoulder posture by gliding your shoulder blades on top of your mid back.

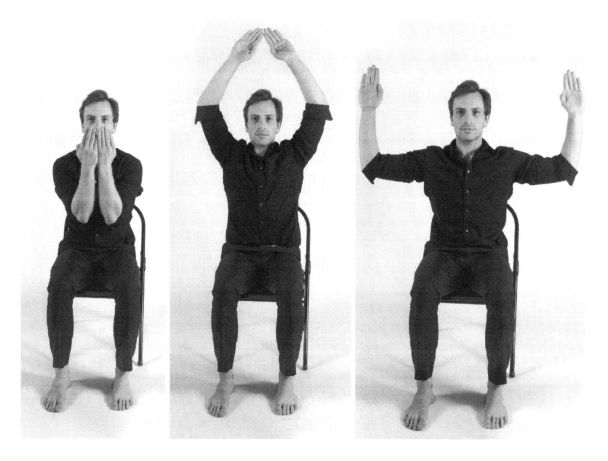

Video 36: Seated Angels

Seated Back Arching

Place your hands together over your head like you are preparing to dive and lean backwards, arching over your chair's back rest.

Benefits: This arching motion reverses the rounded lower back posture that occurs from sitting and restores the spines natural curvature, creating an environment for ligament stability.

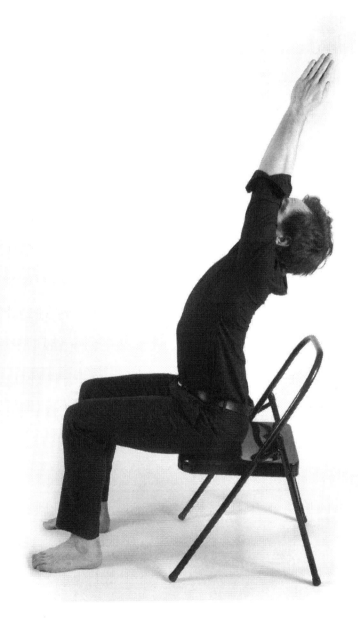

VIDEO 37: SEATED BACK ARCHING

Seated Side-Bends

Raise your arms above your head, bring your palms together, and bend and lift your torso to the left. Switch sides. You should feel a release of tension from your flanks.

Benefits: Side-bending creates an opening and closing effect in the canals where the nerve roots exit the spine, releasing compression and providing a lubricated effect to the rib cage region and diaphragm. This makes the move especially useful for those of you who sit in one position every day, day after day.

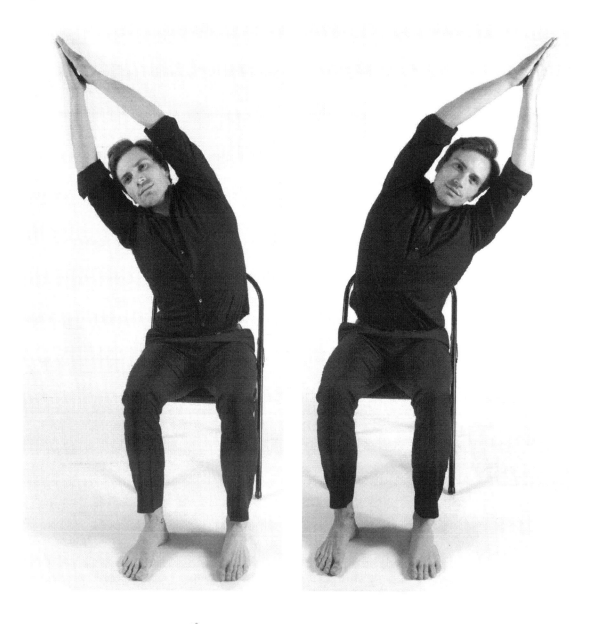

VIDEO 38: SEATED SIDE BENDS

Seated Golf Twists

Cross your arms over your chest and try to keep your head straight while you twist the rib cage left and right to a comfortable position. As you move, you'll find that your range of motion improves.

Benefits: These twists improve the range of motion of your rib cage at the thoracic wall and send excitatory messages to the spinal rotators to help wake them up. It's as if they are piano keys being played up and down the spine, trying to provide information about your body to its environment. This is called proprioception, and, as we age, we lose proprioception. This exercise is great to retrain our bodies for longevity.

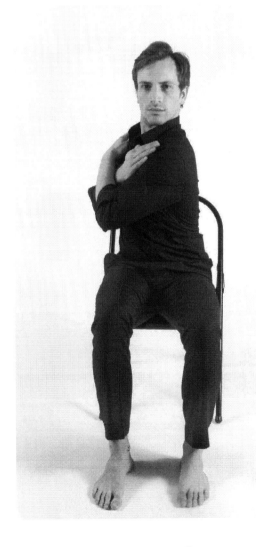 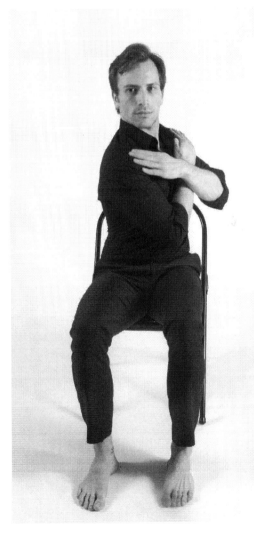

VIDEO 39: SEATED GOLF TWISTS

Seated Posture Reset

Sit on the edge of your chair, tuck your feet in and under toward your buttocks, squeeze your shoulder blades back and down, and pull your head on top of your shoulders. Essentially, give yourself a double chin—or that's the effect anyway. You should feel tension build in the back of your shoulders and your middle back. This is another one of my go-to exercises for perfect posture.

Benefits: This exercise takes the load of your head (which weighs about 10–15 lbs) and places it in a neutral plane on top of your spine. This eases head, neck, and upper back tension, which is essential to reduce lower back strain while in a seated posture. This movement also teaches your middle back to hold your shoulder blades inward and down, helping prevent rounded shoulder and rounded (Kyphotic) upper back posture. Rounded upper back postures place excessive strain to the lower spine. Its essential to correct this in order to alleviate lower back problems. Side note: This movement is excellent for relieving head and neck pain (maybe we will cover that in my next book).

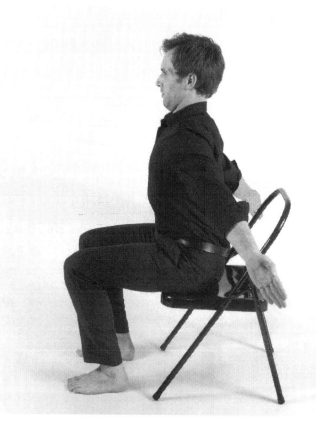

📹 **Video 40: Seated Posture Reset**

Seated Hip Closers and Openers*

Cross your leg with your knee high, clasp that knee with your hands, and pull toward opposite shoulder. You should feel tension stretching through the outer hip (i.e., your sciatic muscle). Next, cross your ankle over the opposite knee, pushing your knee down with one hand and holding your ankle with the other. Repeat on the other side. You should feel tension release from your inner thigh and groin.

Benefits: This action helps provide motion to the hip sockets and provides synovial fluid to the ball and socket joints. In this way, it prevents adhesions and the buildup of scar tissue in the hip joint that limits mobility and leads to the onset of arthritis. Designed to take the pressure off the sciatic notch muscles of your hip, this exercise alleviates deep buttocks, lower back, and sciatic nerve tightening. Compression from the act of sitting is known to irritate the sciatic nerve.

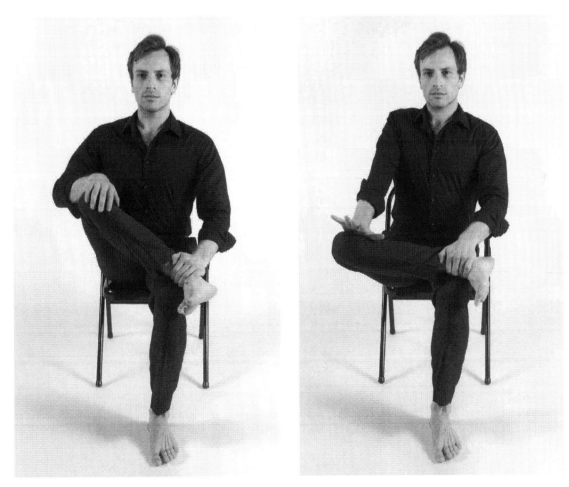

*AVOID THESE IF YOU'VE HAD A HIP OR KNEE REPLACEMENT.

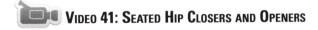 VIDEO 41: SEATED HIP CLOSERS AND OPENERS

Seated Back Traction*

While seated in a chair, try to brace your upper body on your armrests, letting your pelvis and legs dangle. You should feel pressure release from your mid and lower back. It's a convenient way to reduce lower back compression without fancy equipment.

Benefits: By using your body weight, the weight of the pelvis creates a traction force, which safely decompresses and releases spinal compression that builds from a seated posture.

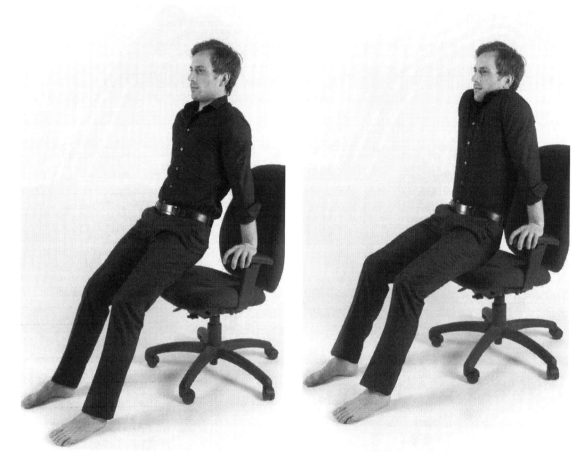

*AVOID IF YOUR CHAIR HAS ROLLERS AND IS ON A SLIPPERY SURFACE

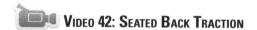 VIDEO 42: SEATED BACK TRACTION

Workday Tension Standing Routine

Time commitment: 60–90 seconds
(Hold each of these movements for 10 seconds every time you stand up)

Standing Back Arch

Reverse the effects of sitting. With your hands on your upper buttocks, stretch backwards from your waist with your feet together. You should feel tension release in the small of your back and lower part of your upper back.

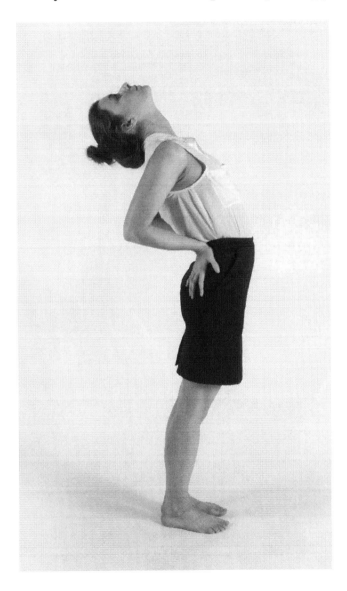

VIDEO 43: STANDING BACK ARCH

Lunge and Reach

Lunge forward with your left hand extended up and your left leg behind you, squeeze the glute of your rear leg and simultaneously lift your rib cage upward and breathe deep to enhance the movement. Repeat on the opposite side. You should feel a release of tension through the upper thigh and rib cage.

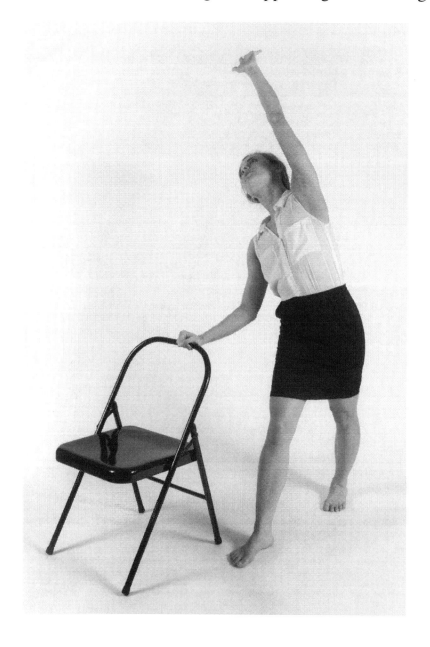

VIDEO 44: LUNGE AND REACH

Sky Reaches

Place your right hand on your left wrist and stretch your left hand up. Cross your left leg behind your right leg and bend to the side. Try to lift your ribcage toward the ceiling and breathe inward to release pressure from your diaphragm. Repeat on the opposite side. You should feel a release of tension in your hips and waist.

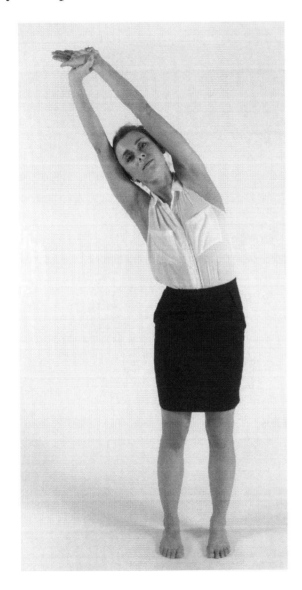
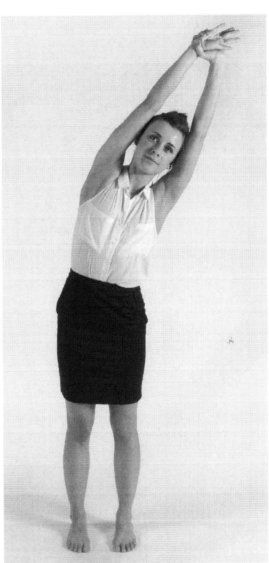

Diving Archer

Stand up and reach your arms over your head, touching your palms together. Arch backwards, leading with your hands. You should feel release of tension in your lower back.

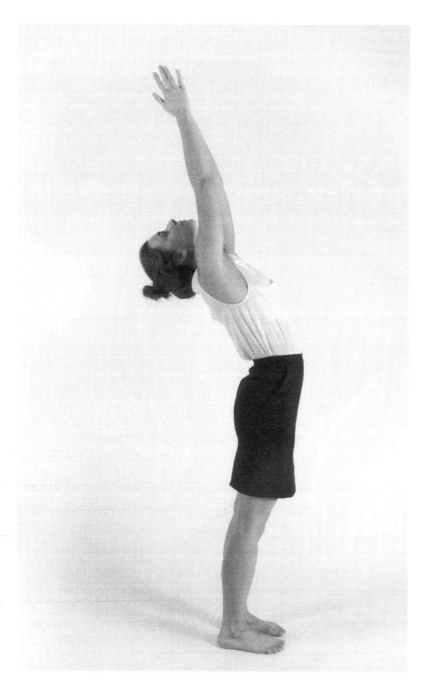

VIDEO 45: DIVING ARCHER

Standing Pelvic Thrusts

Standing still, sway your lower back and then flatten it. You should feel a release of tension from the lower back. With your feet shoulder-width apart, fold your arms across your chest, tuck your belly button in toward your spine, and tuck in your pelvis. This movement helps lubricate the lower spinal facet joints. Then reverse the motion by arching your back. This anterior to posterior gliding movement exaggerates a sway back and then transitions to a pelvic tuck or flat back.

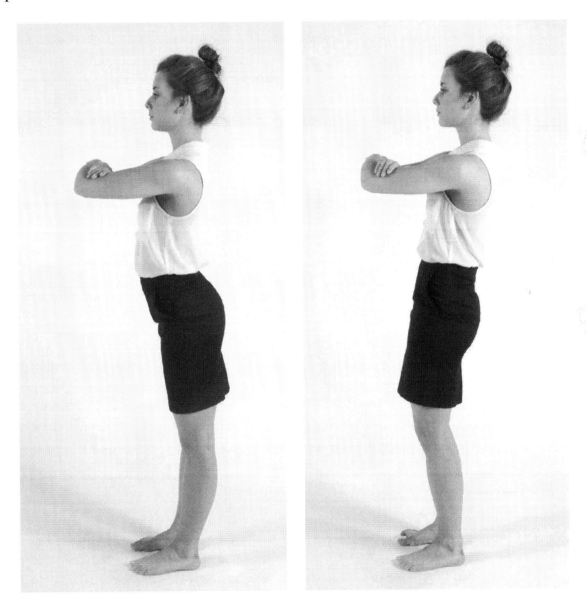

VIDEO 46: STANDING PELVIC THRUSTS

Golf Twists

With your feet shoulder-width apart, fold your arms across your chest while keeping your head facing forward and twist your body from side to side. This targets the mid back.

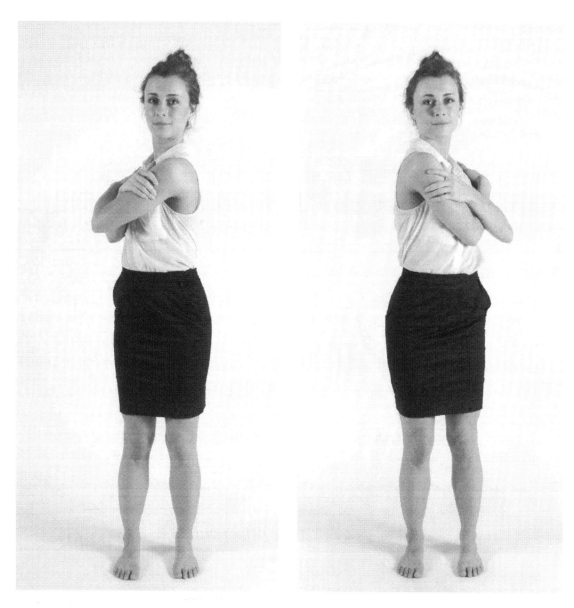

VIDEO 47: GOLF TWISTS

Standing Pelvic Twists

Cross your arms in front of you at shoulder level and twist from left to right with your pelvis, moving the bottom half of your torso and legs with each twist. The emphasis should be on keeping your upper body still. Furthermore, you may hear and feel a release from the upper portion of your lower back. The release from the upper portion of your lower back creates a sense of mobility and separation/proprioception awareness. Joints between the lower back and pelvis are also lubricated with this motion

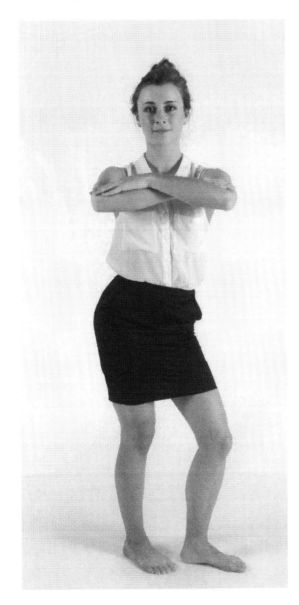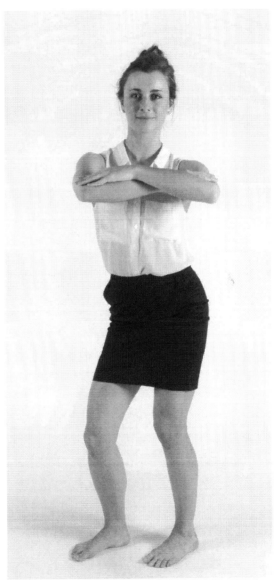

VIDEO 48: STANDING PELVIC TWISTS

Standing Pelvic Clocks

Stand like you would for pelvic twists with your feet shoulder-width apart, then slowly move your hips and pelvis as if you were playing with a hula hoop, slowly gyrating your belly button in a circular pattern. Think of the dances at a Hawaiian luau. This is a 3-dimensional way to lubricate your spine.

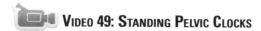 VIDEO 49: STANDING PELVIC CLOCKS

Hacky Sack

Standing upright, try to touch your ankle to your opposite hand. This movement is similar to kicking a ball with the inner sole of your foot. This activates your hip rotators and helps prevent sciatica.

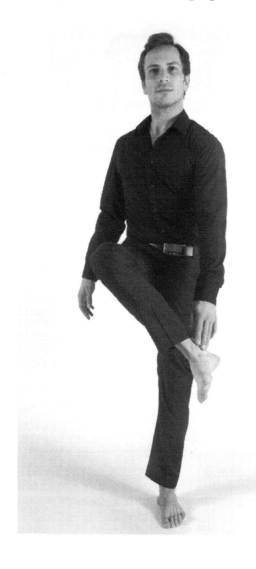 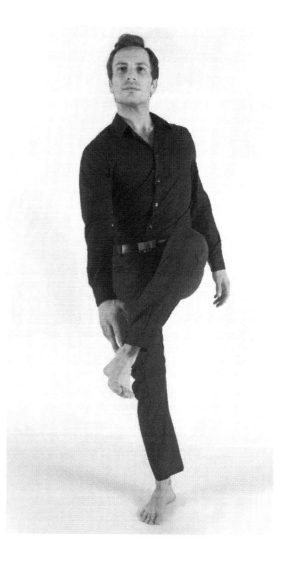

VIDEO 50: HACKY SACK

Counter Traction*

Find a stable countertop that is about waist high and support your upper body on it while allowing your legs to dangle. You should feel a release of pressure from your mid to lower back.

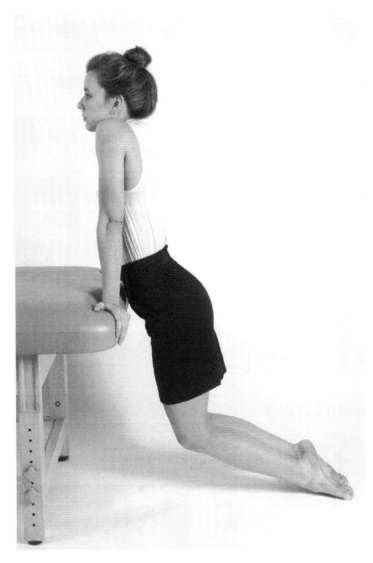

*AVOID IF YOU HAVE SHOULDER PROBLEMS

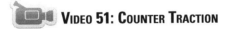 VIDEO 51: COUNTER TRACTION

What If You Stand All Day at Work?

Try to do the opposite of someone who sits all day; sit whenever possible to take the load off. Once you get a chance to sit down, perform the seated chair routines. You have an advantage over people who sit at work—you can move more easily and consistently throughout the day. If you're in a safe environment, perform the standing movement routine listed on page 49 whenever possible.

Avoid the temptation to stretch out your back. The truth is, despite the fact that you stand all day, you probably bend, stoop, and lift during your occupation, placing undue stress and tension on your spine. Take the load off and sit, but avoid stretching out your back. It may already be weakened and vulnerable to injury. Remember, most back attacks happen while bending forward in flexion when performing activities you've done thousands of times before, like bending forward to tie your shoes.

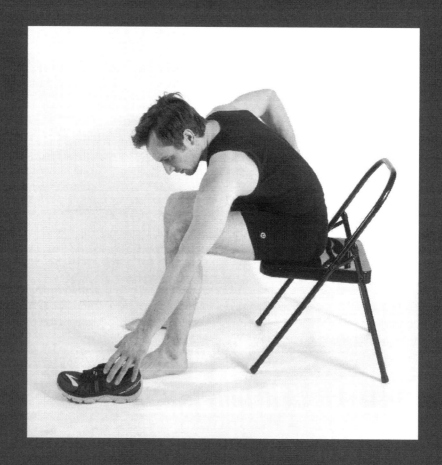

Evening Decompression Routines

So far, so good. You know what to do in the morning, you know what to do at work. Now, you're home and you need to take the load off your back. It doesn't matter if you stand or sit all day. What matters is how to decompress your spine so that it's not jammed up before you go to sleep at night. During the course of the day, our spine compresses and changes shape. We need to control the effects of gravity and prevent the onset of arthritis and degeneration associated with spinal compression.

Think of it as a loaded, compressed spring being pulled apart. The following postures are simple to apply and will help result in a more evenly balanced spinal load by alleviating pressure from one particular region of the lower back, and essentially creating an even distribution to share the load. So get comfortable, put on loose clothing, and perform the following exercises.

Uncoiling the Spine—If You Sit All Day

Time commitment: 5 minutes

Modified Cobra*

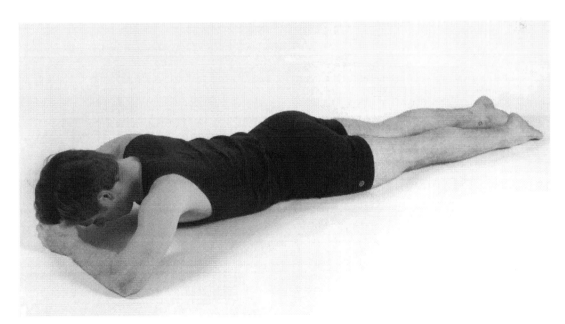

* Note: Avoid this posture if you have spondylolisthesis.

These exercises reset your lumbar or low back curve. If you sit all day, your low back loses it natural curve and the discs leak fluid backwards toward your spinal canal. So, when home, reverse this process by resetting your arch. This posture will offset the effects of sitting by restoring a natural curve to the low back. Do not over exert; simply lay face down and relax. Your joints will relax, decompress the pressure of the discs, and slowly uncoil. Do not extend or over arch your back.

Uncoiling the Spine—If You Stand All Day

Time commitment: 10 minutes

The Ottoman

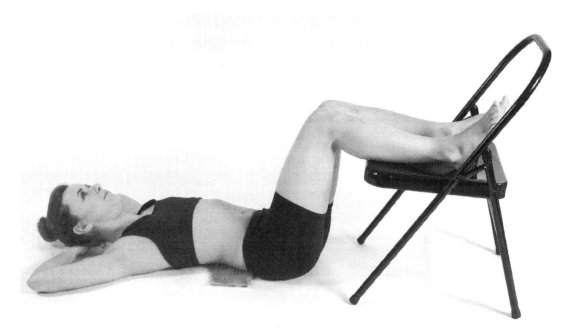

Adopting the posture shown here after standing all day will give your low back a chance to decompress, uncoiling the compression and jamming of the low back joints associated with standing. Simply put your feet up, lie on your back, and just stay there for 10 minutes. This is the minimum amount of time proven to equilibrate and redistribute spinal disc pressure and take the compression off spine sensitive structures like nerves and joints.

Use ice under the small of the lower back while in the Ottoman posture if your intention is to reduce swelling. This, of course, is optional, but if you choose to use ice, make sure to place a barrier between you and the ice pack to prevent an ice burn.

Evening Decompression Floor Routine

Time commitment: 5 minutes

Here is a set of additional movements to help uncoil your back, whether you sit or stand all day. The evening floor routine is identical to the morning floor routine. I review the movements here for your convenience.

Hip Drops

On your back, lift your legs in the air as if you're sitting in a chair. Keeping your arms out to the side for balance, drop your hips from side to side. Perform until your feet are against the floor.

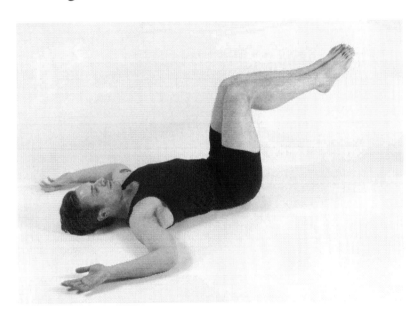

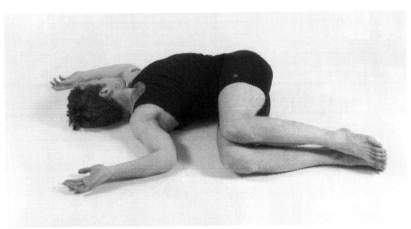

📹 **VIDEO 18: HIP DROPS**

Recumbent Pelvic Tilts

While lying on your back, try to exaggerate the sway of the lower back curve, then flatten out the curvature and repeat, moving back and forth until limber.

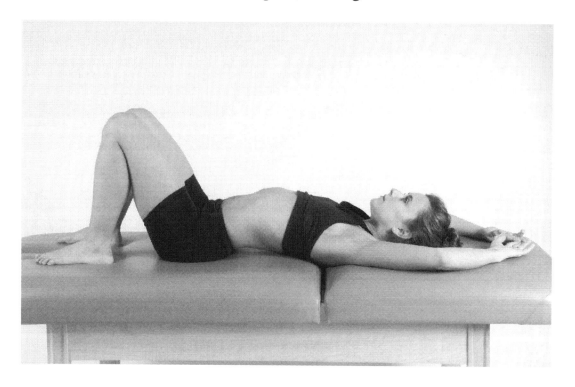

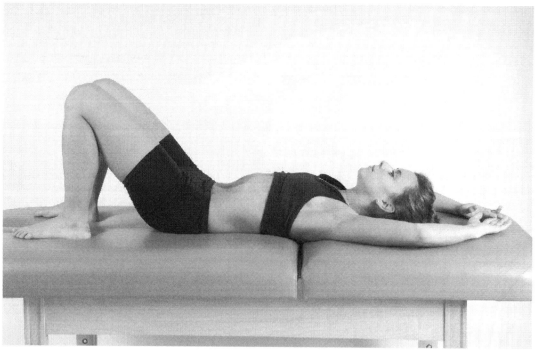

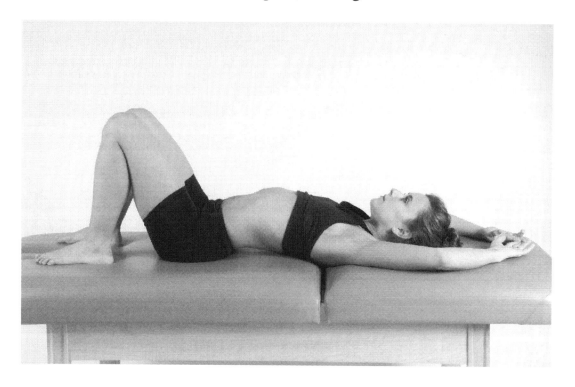 **VIDEO 52: RECUMBENT PELVIC TILTS**

Hip Openers*

Lie on your back, bend both knees, keeping your feet on the floor, and cross one ankle over the other knee. Take your hand and gently push and pull the knee of the crossed ankle in and out.

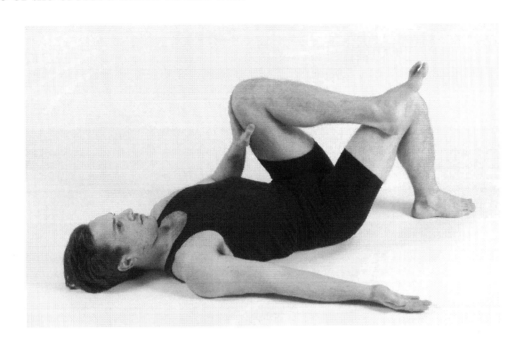

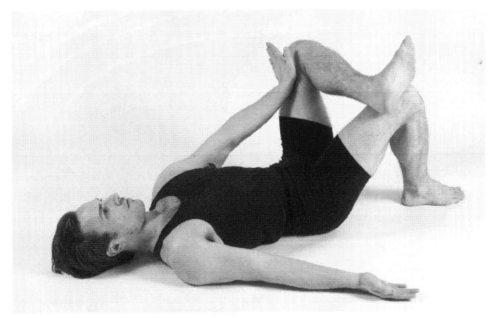

*AVOID THIS EXERCISE IF YOU HAVE A HIP REPLACEMENT.

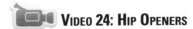 VIDEO 24: HIP OPENERS

Dynamic Hamstrings

On your back, with your knees bent and feet on the floor, grab your right thigh with both hands and then straighten and bend your knee repeatedly. Repeat with the left thigh.

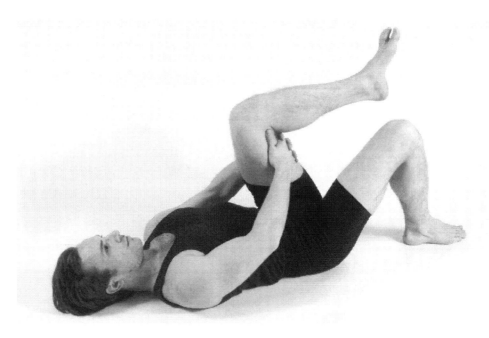

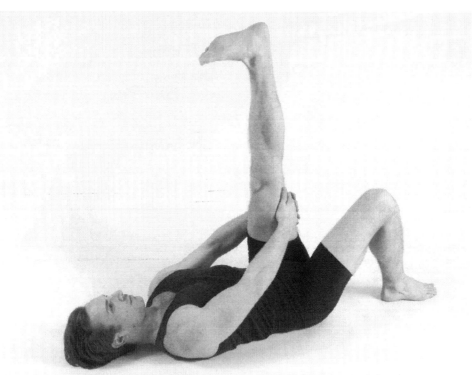

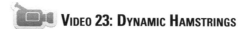 VIDEO 23: DYNAMIC HAMSTRINGS

Dynamic Hip Flexors*

Lie down on your side and pull the bottom leg up toward your chest. Use the top arm to grab the top foot/knee (hold wherever is most comfortable for you). Flex your knee and thigh to your chest, then try to pull your heel to your buttock.

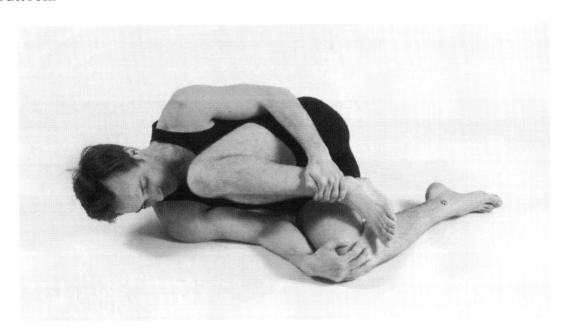

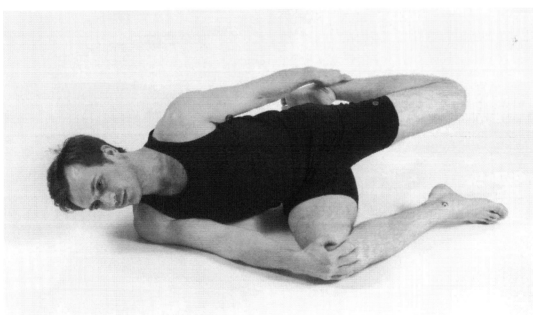

*AVOID THIS EXERCISE IF YOU HAVE HIP OR KNEE REPLACEMENTS

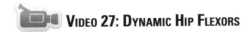 VIDEO 27: DYNAMIC HIP FLEXORS

Open Books

Lie on your side in a fetal position with your arms straight out in front. Open up your body like you would a book, making sure to keep your legs on the floor while twisting the torso.

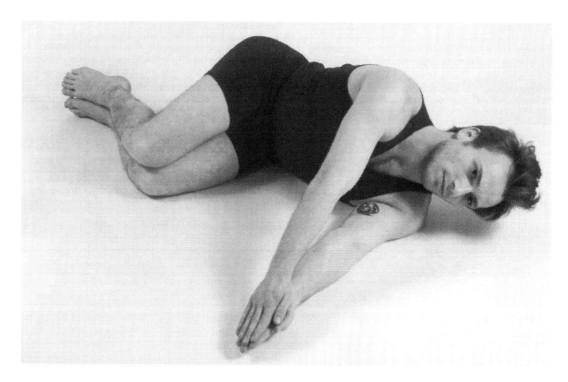

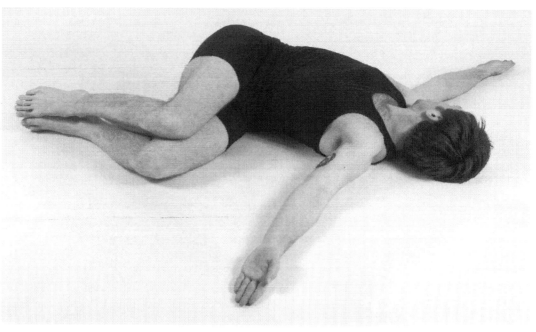

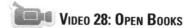 **VIDEO 28: OPEN BOOKS**

Modified Cobra on Forearms*

This is an exercise meant to extend and slightly exaggerate the curvature of the lower back. Resting your head while lying on your stomach is usually intended as a spinal decompression stretch; however, here it is meant to exaggerate the arch by pushing upward on your forearms. Again, don't tighten your low back muscles, just relax into this posture.

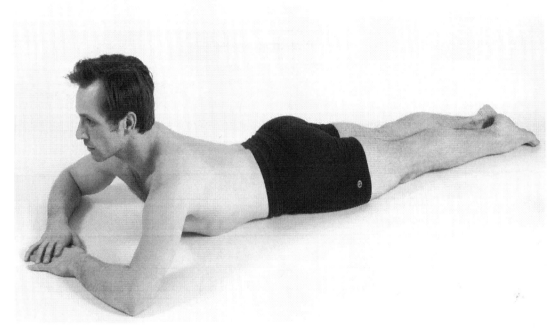

*AVOID IF YOU HAVE AN EXAGGERATED ARCH IN YOUR LOWER BACK OR IF YOU HAVE SPONDYLOLISTHESIS

Reach-Backs

On all fours, place one hand behind your head and reach down, touching your elbow to the inside of your straight arm. Then, reach in the opposite direction by pointing your elbow toward the ceiling, let your gaze follow your moving arm.

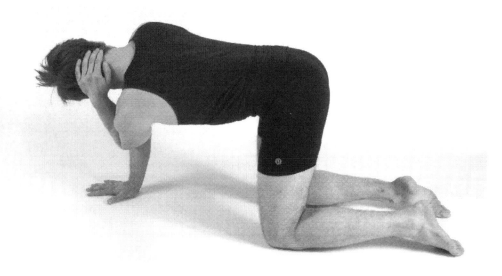

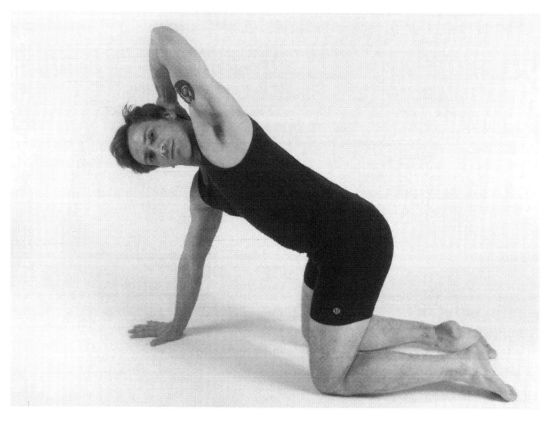

🎥 Video 32: Reach-Backs

Cat and Cow

On all fours, round your back and drop your head forward. Reverse the action by arching your back and extending your head to look up at the ceiling. Focus on flaring and pinching your shoulder blades as you move.

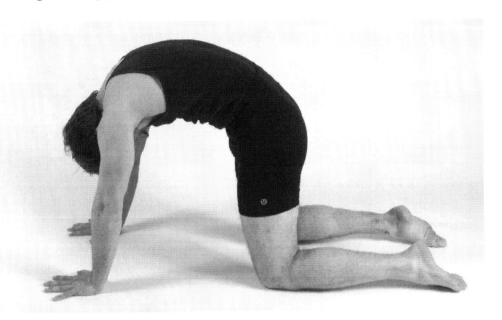

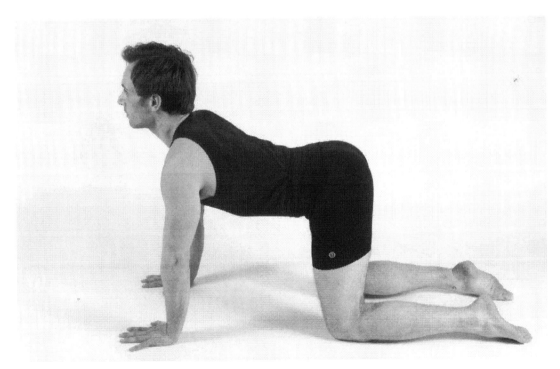

VIDEO 34: CAT AND COW

Abdominal Brace and Stand

Now brace and stand up. Ending with this movement sequence ensures you lock in the benefits of the routine.

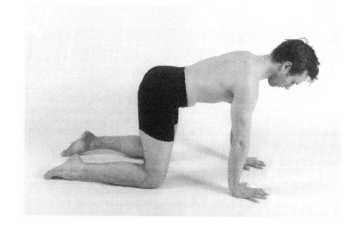

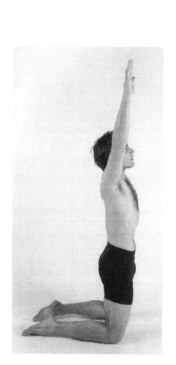
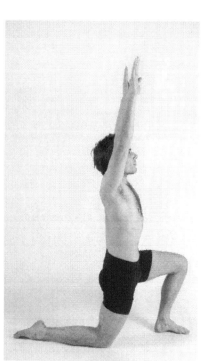
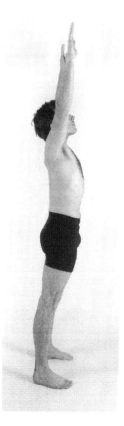

VIDEO 2: KNEELING TO STANDING ABDOMINAL BRACING

Congratulations! You are ready to end your day.

Daily Stretch Routine: The Five Essential Stretches

Time commitment: 5 minutes
(hold each stretch for 15 seconds, twice on each side)

Okay, here are the good stretches I promised to share with you. They relieve pressure from your spine without having to target your back muscles directly. These moves are extremely safe and effective because they aid the postural muscles to help keep your spine erect. These muscles shorten and tighten from the seated and long-standing postures that are often adopted throughout the work day.

I prefer that you perform these stretches each evening just prior to bedtime, that way you can stretch out all those short, tight muscles after a full day of supporting your posture. Better yet, you can set yourself up for a restful night's sleep and the likelihood of waking up in the morning a little more limber. If you have had a joint replacement to your hip or knee, I have provided an alternate routine with recommended ways to achieve the effectiveness of these stretches. However, you should also show your surgeon the exercises beforehand and ask for permission to do these movements. They know your individual case better than anyone.

Side Stretch

While standing, place your legs wide apart. Bring one arm overhead and reach towards the other side and upwards to the ceiling. While concentrating on lifting the rib cage, take a deep breath in to activate the attachments to your diaphragm, then cross the leg on the same side as the lifted arm behind the other leg.

Anatomy: Quadratus lumborum, tensor fasciae latae, abdominal oblique

Benefits: The muscles involved in this exercise have a tendency to cramp during the day and, when they shorten, will create a hip hiking, which results in a functional short leg. This biomechanical flaw will shear tension on the spine. These muscles are generally involved with disc herniation injuries, especially to the quadratus luborum as it attaches directly to the pelvis, moves to the rib cage, then takes a right angle turn and attaches to the spine. It wreaks havoc on low back pain sufferers. Therefore, this is a great stretch for your waist, rib cage, and outer thigh.

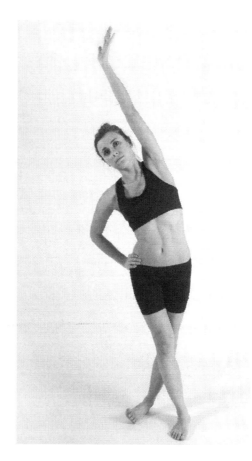

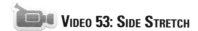 **Video 53: Side Stretch**

Lunge Stretch

Use an elevated surface like a couch, a massage table, or your bed. Take a stance as if you're a fencer and place the rear leg on the elevated bed surface. Then, lunge forward deeper, making sure your front leg keeps a 90-degree angle. Helpful hint: keep your kneecap in alignment with your heel; do not move your knee forward on top of your toes. This is a two-part stretch. Once in the posture, try and tighten your glutes. When you do this, you'll feel a stretch to the front of your thigh. This feeling should make you aware of what we are trying to stretch. Then try to grab your back ankle and bring your heel toward your butt.

Anatomy: Psoas, iliacus, quadriceps (commonly known as the hip flexors)

Benefits: The hip flexors attach the front of your hip and pelvis to the entire lumbar spine. When short and tight (from the act of a seated posture or years of incorrect sit ups, etc.) this muscle group will tug your lower back forward, creating a sway-back posture that will consequently jam the facet joints together. Essentially, you're squashing them and the discs between. This stretch, like the others, is essential to relieving lower back pain.

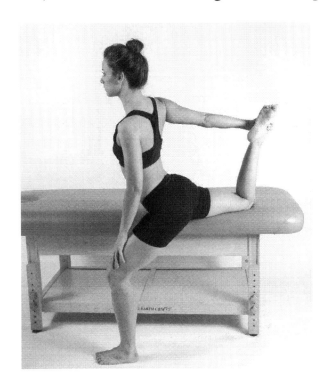

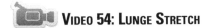 **VIDEO 54: LUNGE STRETCH**

Hip Rotator Stretch

Using a bed or couch for elevation, bend one knee to 90 degrees, then place it flat on the surface. Lunge your other leg backwards, and then bend your back knee, creating the motion of sitting. Lean forward on top of your thigh.

Anatomy: Piriformis, gluteus medius, and other small rotators of the hip.

Benefits: The above muscles tighten just with the act of walking. They also shorten when inactive or compressed by sitting. Due to their anatomical orientation, when dysfunctional, they affect the sciatic nerve. If you have had a hip replacement, they have probably been short and tight for many years. They attach your hip to the sacrum, which is the base of the spine. If one side is tighter than the other, it can pull on the sacrum, causing sacroiliac instability, which will tilt your pelvis and shear your spine. Again, this is a must in the world of stretching to relieve lower back pain. This is a great stretch for the front of your buttocks, outer hip, and thigh.

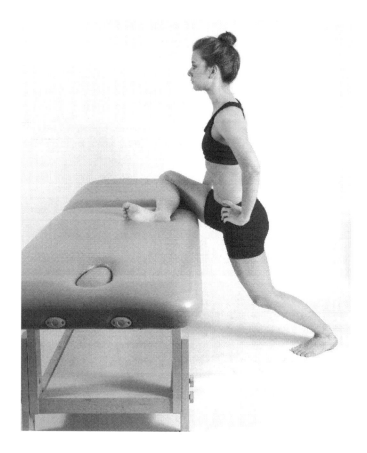

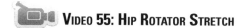 **VIDEO 55: HIP ROTATOR STRETCH**

Hamstring Stretch

Use a bed or couch and keep a neutral low back posture (meaning don't over arch or flatten your back while performing this stretch). Place one leg on top of the surface, flex your foot by pointing your toes toward your head, and then gently hinge at the waist, keeping your lower back straight.

Note:

1. If your bed is too high, your knee will bend and the stretch is ineffective, so use a lower bench, chair, or stool.
2. Do not round the lower back; keep it arched or as straight as possible and, for goodness sake, don't try to flatten it.

Anatomy: Hamstrings, calves, and adductors

Benefits: My clinical observations lead me to believe that most low-back-pain sufferers have shortened hamstrings. Anatomically, the hamstrings will flatten the lower back when short and tight. Furthermore, the facet joints are meant to prevent excessive movement of the spine, like hinges that monitor motion. When you have a flattened curve, the facet joints lose their functionality and excessive motion occurs prematurely, wearing out the joints. Over time, the spine tries to compensate by providing stability with the laying down of calcium as a way to fuse or stop hyper-mobility. Degenerative changes to the discs start occurring because of a lack of mobility and calcium deposits. All of this crowds the spinal canal, causing spinal stenosis (a clogging of the spinal canal) and probable cord compression. The most challenging lower back condition to heal is when someone has lost his or her natural curvature because the spinal load is now being placed vertically and is no longer dispersed evenly on the disc spaces. This is why this stretch is so important. I have found that by simultaneously limbering the insertion behind both the knees and the buttocks area, you'll release tension to the entire muscle and help stop the progression of a flat back posture.

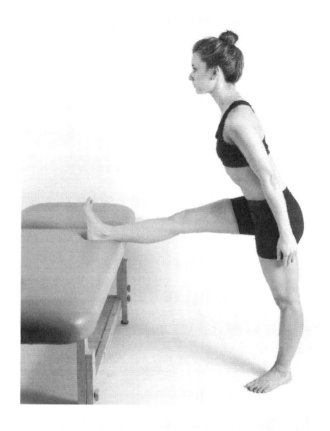

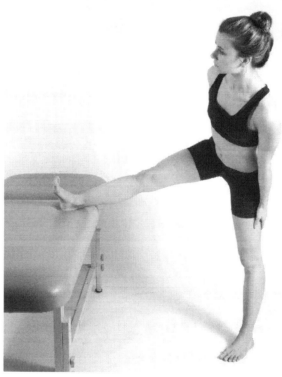

VIDEO **56**: HAMSTRING STRETCH

Full Spine Stretch

Unless you have balance problems, you can use a bed or couch for elevation in this stretch. Lie on your side, bend your bottom hip and knee, and keep your top hip stacked on top of the bottom hip. Keep the top knee straight and slightly extended behind you, preferably hanging off the bed. Then, while keeping your lower body still, try to rotate your upper torso so that you are lying chest-down on the bed. Breathe deeply and you should feel a release of tension in your diaphragm, front of the pelvis, and lower back.

Anatomy: Erector spinae, multifidi rotators, abdominal obliques

Benefits: This is a full spinal stretch involving the entire biomechanical chain from your torso to your feet. There is very low spinal loading while you achieve full mobility to the entire spine. You target the spinal rotators at the same time as the spinal erectors, pelvic hip flexors, abductors, and abdominal muscles. All these areas communicate when we move, so why not stretch and challenge them all at the same time, just like normal daily movements. This stretch is a great way to tie it all in together.

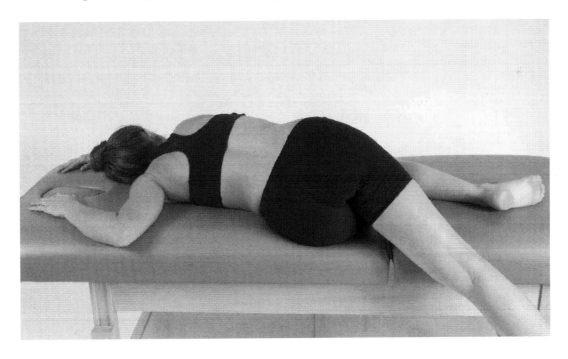

VIDEO 57: FULL SPINE STRETCH

Alternate Stretch Routine for Hip and Knee Replacements and Injuries

Hanging Thigh Stretch

Lie face up on your bed, slide to the edge, and let one leg drop towards the floor. Hold your other thigh at 90 degrees—you'll feel a great stretch to the front of your thigh.

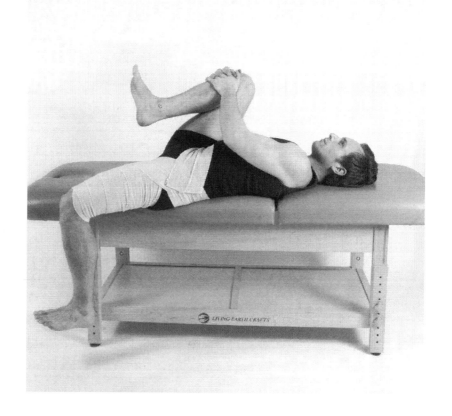

VIDEO 58: HANGING THIGH STRETCH

Standing Lunge Stretch

Simply stand upright and lunge the surgical leg backwards. Raise the same arm as your surgical leg above your head and tilt sideways. Now, squeeze your buttocks and press your heel to the floor. You'll feel a great stretch to the front of your thigh and by tilting sideways your fully stretch the hip.

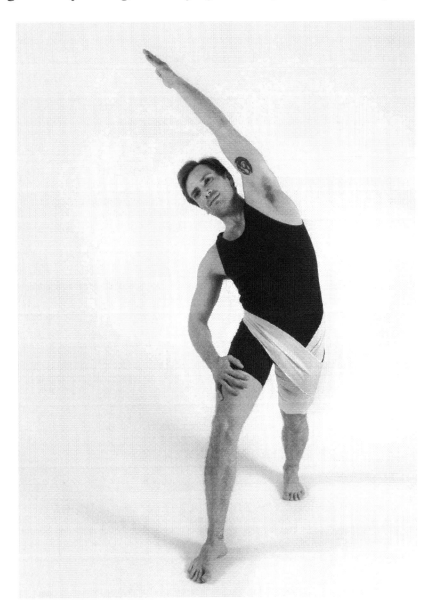

VIDEO 60: STANDING LUNGE STRETCH

Lunge Against a Chair Stretch

While standing, lean on a chair and simply lunge your surgical leg backwards, keeping it straight. Try and press your heel to the floor, then squeeze your buttocks. Squeezing the buttocks will create a greater stretch to the front of your thigh. Then lean to the opposite side to ensure a full hip flexor stretch.

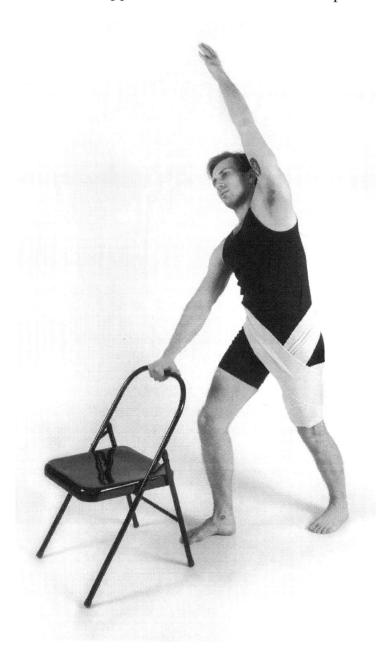

VIDEO 59: LUNGE ON A STOOL STRETCH

Side Lying Hip Rotator Stretch

Using a bed or couch for elevation, lie on your nonsurgical side and bring your surgical leg halfway up toward your chest. Next, bend your knee about 90 degrees, then gently, with the buttocks, try to drop that ankle towards the floor to generate a greater stretch.

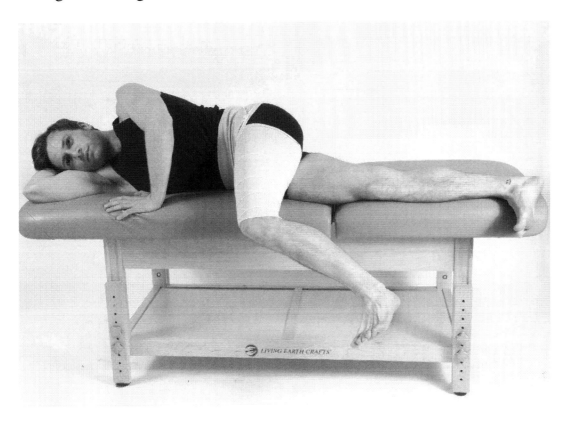

VIDEO 61: SIDE LYING HIP ROTATOR STRETCH

Awaken Your Core from Amnesia

When people talk about the core, they traditionally think of performing sit-ups and crunches to strengthen their abs. This is completely outdated and essentially harmful, as already discussed. The core refers to all the muscles of your trunk, which supports your spine. There are 29 pairs in all that connect the low back to the hips, pelvis, and rib cage. Think of your core exercises as building a corset, a brace which surrounds your low back all the way around, rather than just a concentration of ab curls and back-arching exercises.

The core runs from the front → flank → rear → other flank → back to the front again. When you think of the core, think of a hoop of connecting architecture (see Diagram 5).

Say someone told you a fairy tale about performing one exercise that cured lower back pain forever. Of course you'd try it. Who wouldn't?

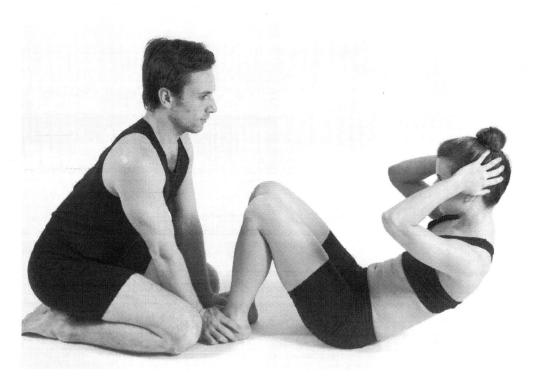

The problem is you're only developing strength in one area.

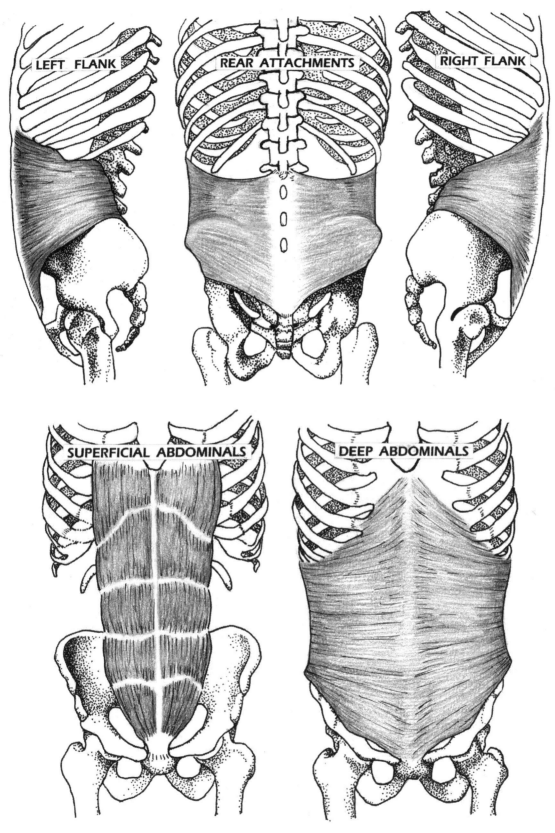

LEFT FLANK

REAR ATTACHMENTS

RIGHT FLANK

SUPERFICIAL ABDOMINALS

DEEP ABDOMINALS

Diagram 5: Core architecture

Your core is 3-D. Each part connects to the next. If you leave out one or more sides while exercising, you're training your back to give out and buckle. In 1961, researchers revealed that 20 pounds is the maximum compression an unsupported spine (a spine with no muscles bracing it) can handle without buckling. Only 20 lbs! Its clear that strength is not the issue when it comes to core stabilization. Here's the analogy (as described by Dr. Stuart McGill, the foremost spinal biomechanics specialist in the world): take a pole, stand the pole upright, and apply a slight downward pressure so that it easily buckles. That is what will happen to your back if you do not exercise all the muscles which surround your core.

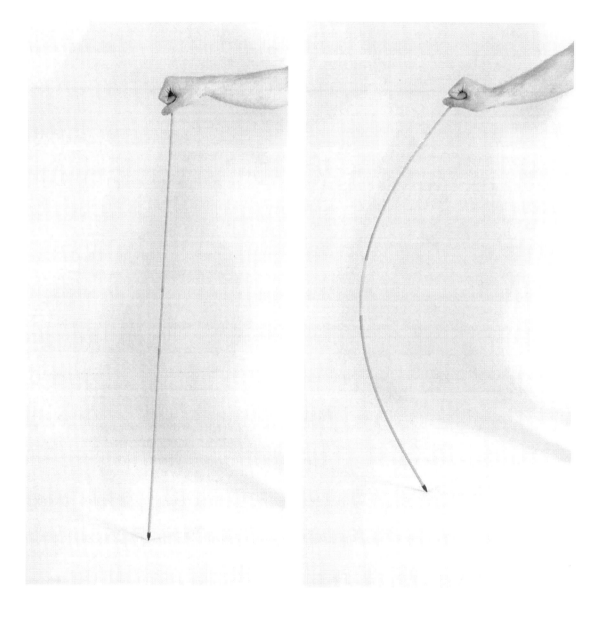

Now, take that same pole, attach guy wires at different heights along its length, and insert them into the ground in a circle as though you were pitching a tent. Pull each wire with a similar tension. Now, if you compress as before, the pole can withstand the force. But reduce the tension in just one wire and the pole will buckle. This is similar to what happens to the spine: the pole is your spine and the wires are your muscles, and when they co-contract, this means they are all active at the same time. This ensures that the spine will not buckle in a similar way, as abdominal bracing is done with daily tasks. As with a symphony, when one instrument is out of tune, the sound is distorted. When a spinal torso muscle loses its ability to engage, the whole spine can fail. Everything has to work together, in concert, like an orchestra. If one group of muscles is not developed, another must take up the slack. Soon, those groups of muscles that are forced to work overtime exceed what they are designed to do, become overloaded, and fail. The other groups become even weaker or atrophied and a domino effect begins. This causes a cascade of spinal failures, which over time lead to low back pain and recurrent injury.

Ever bend forward to pick up a light item off the floor—say a pencil or a shoe—and you throw your back out? Was the pencil heavy? Were your knees bent? Was your back straight? Honestly, who cares? You've performed this movement thousands of times before. Why did your back buckle now? It all has to do with your core muscles working in unison. If one side is weak or activates out of sync, then faulty motor patterns develop, placing stress on the spine and eventually leading to injuries to the low back—like the straw that broke the camel's back.

Research dictates that only 10% of your torso muscles need to be coactivated at any one time to ensure spine stability during most daily tasks, such as getting dressed, grooming, opening doors, changing postures from sitting to standing, and so on. It's even enough to protect you from sudden slips or falls.

Thus, it would appear that your strength has very little to do with protecting your back. You see, you don't need to be a body builder to strengthen your spine. On the contrary, all you need to do is wake up your spinal core muscles from amnesia. Train them to be active, only 10% active, all day; this way, when needed, they can protect your spine from the daily stresses placed upon it.

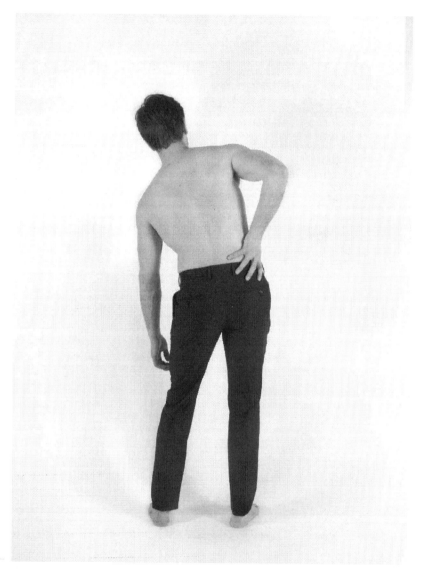

Even picking up a penny can cause your back to buckle if one side of your core is weak.

Core Endurance

Core endurance is the ability to maintain a low level of support all day to stabilize your spine during daily activities. Studies show that reduced spinal erector endurance is a predictor for future risk of low back trouble and that muscle endurance is more important than strength when it comes to the lower back. The more core endurance you have, the less likely it is that you will have back pain. It's not about how much weight you can lift; it's about how long you can hold a neutral spine posture. The longer you can do this, the healthier your back is. The less time you can hold the posture, the more likely you will have back pain. If your core muscle groups cannot hold your posture upright for long periods of time, you're a person who is at risk for future back pain.

Interpreting the Data

We know there's a relationship of endurance among the front, flanks, and rear portions of your torso. Once an imbalance occurs, low back trouble begins. I've interpreted the complex and extensive data concerning this and will now try to make it simple for you to understand. Get this part and you'll be one up on hundreds of thousands of people with low back pain.

Remember those guy wires I talked about when pitching a tent? Well, in terms of your spine, each core muscle that acts as a guy wire requires a specific amount of endurance in relation to the others to ensure spine stability.

In terms of endurance, the ratios below have been found to protect your back. Science has shown that in a perfect world, young, healthy individuals (i.e., men and women about 21 years old) should have the following endurance ratios:

1. Your right flank muscles should be 100% equal to your left.
2. Your front abdominal flexor muscles should have about 75% the endurance of your low back extensor muscles.
3. Your flank muscles (either side) should have 50% the endurance of your low back extensor muscles.

The photos that follow are of specific spinal endurance strength tests developed to test the limits of low back endurance. Notice how we test the side flanks, front flexors, and rear extensors. My program is designed to safely build an anatomical corset—a low back brace—with your own muscles. We need to accomplish this without harming your lower back by engaging muscles that do not pull, tug, or shear your spine. These exercises are to be executed without special equipment or weights so that you can perform them easily within the comforts of your own home.

I adopted core posture exercises to mimic the endurance requirements necessary to safely build your anatomical corset. I've taken out all the guesswork and deciphered all the scientific jargon. I have made it easy for you to interpret and execute these exercises to achieve core endurance.

The functional divisions of the abdominal muscles justify the need for several exercise techniques to challenge them. Using time as our guide, we will build endurance to create a lasting anatomical corset that will stabilize our spine. By minimizing harmful spine loading and limiting spinal motion, we will preserve your lower back joints while building strength around them. We will impose low level loads, one side at a time, keeping your low back still and not allowing any movement. We will focus on low level (10% maximum) strength and utilize co-contraction (engaging many muscle groups at once). All exercises will be performed with a neutral spine by keeping your posture in its natural position.

Your breathing pattern is important; *do not hold your breath*. We need to build strength and endurance independent of breathing. Our goal is to establish your anatomical corset so that it is perfectly balanced to support your back during your normal day-to-day activities. Perform all of these exercises in this exact sequence as we update your neurological software.

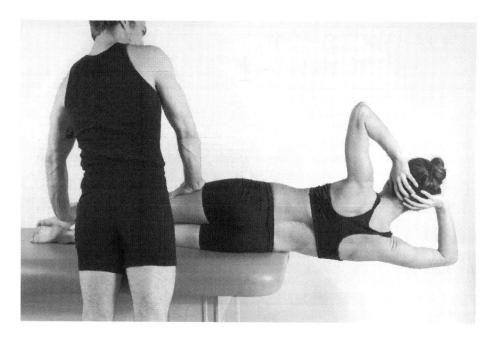

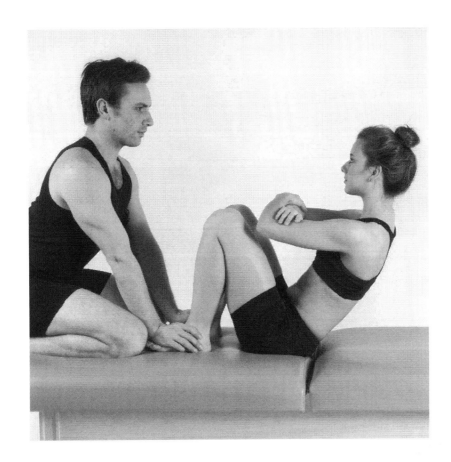

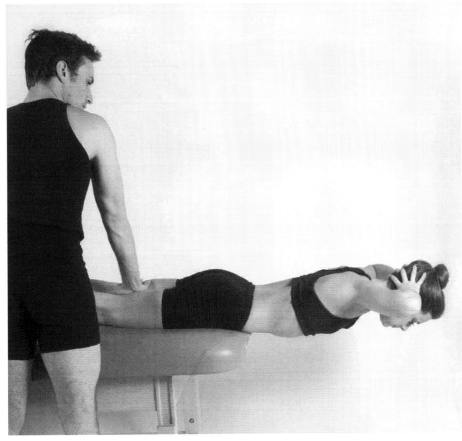

Neck Isometrics

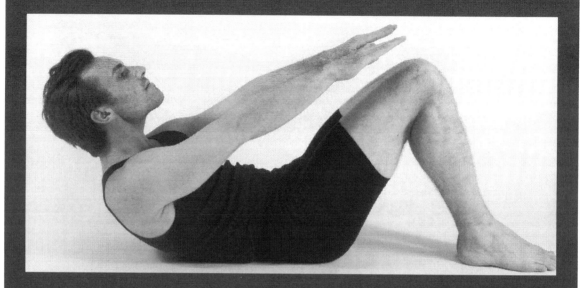

First, while attempting core strengthening, many people strain their neck by jutting the head forward. To prevent neck strain, I advise you to perform these exercises as part of our routine. Isometrics means no movement, so your head stays still as you apply a gentle force on the front, side, and back of your head. Don't hold your breath; breathe in and out independent of force applied. Press against your own pressure, but keep in mind that it's not a strength contest—simply resist your effort gently. The goal is to apply enough pressure that produces an effort of strength but does not overpower your current strength level. This means no movement occurs. And remember, don't hold your breath!

Neck Isometrics (continued)

Hold each exercise for 5 seconds:

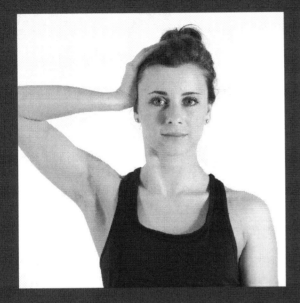 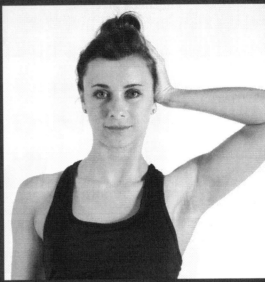

Left and right side isometrics

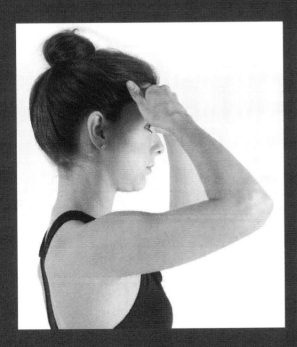 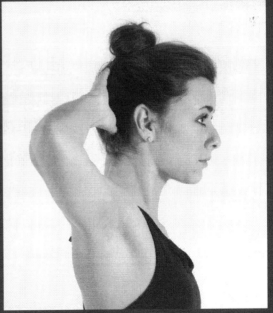

Front and rear side isometrics

Core Endurance Program

Time commitment: 9 minutes

It's important to perform the strength exercises in the exact sequence outlined here. The abdominal muscles fatigue in a strange way, starting with the transverse abdominus, then the abdominal obliques, and finally the rectus abdominus. Since the rectus abdominus assists the motion of all the other abdominal muscles we can not let it fatigue. We need the rectus abdominus to be strong and fresh to help get the most out of the transverse and oblique groups. But don't get too caught up in this, just follow my guidelines. Like I said earlier, I deciphered all the literature to make it easy and less confusing. I am certain the complexity of the information is a reason why low back pain is still an enormous problem for most people. It's science, dude!

Front Plank (Advanced exercise, good for athletic people)

While in a military push-up position and keeping a neutral spine, rest your upper body weight on your forearms, keep your abdominals engaged and tucked in, and don't let your lower back sag towards the floor. Here, we are training the co-activation of the abdominals, hip flexors, and low back erectors all at the same time. By limiting movement, we achieve spinal stability. Now, work on endurance.

Primary muscles trained: Transverse abdominals, hip flexors, and spinal erectors.

Goal: 90 seconds. Perform once or use multiple sets to achieve goal (e.g., 9 reps for 10 seconds each).

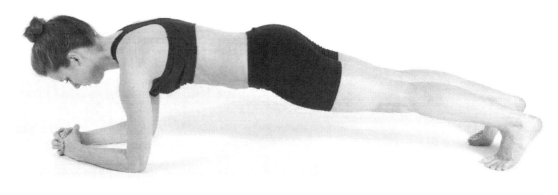

VIDEO 62: FRONT PLANK

Half plank

If a full plank is too challenging, start with a half plank (good for beginners). Balance on your forearms and, instead of balancing on your toes, balance on your knees. Put a cushion under your knees to prevent compression of your kneecaps.

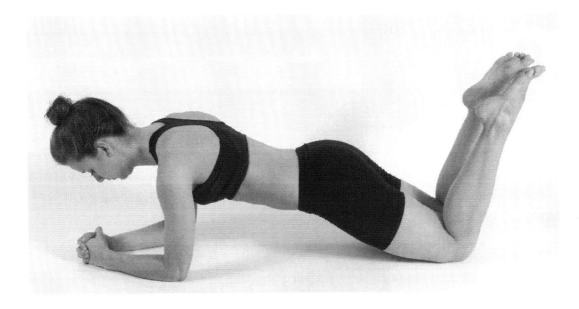

VIDEO 63: HALF PLANK

Single-Leg Back Bridge
(Advanced exercise, good for athletic people)

Lie on your back with both knees bent and your feet on the floor. Activate all abdominal muscles. Do not flatten the lower back but keep it in a curve by maintaining a neutral spine. Lift your pelvis up until your thighs are in line with your waist. Next, straighten out one knee and flex your toes upward. Avoid excessive sway back arching while performing this exercise. We are trying to engage both the glutes and spinal erectors while challenging the abdominal muscles. We are creating our muscular hoop. Remember, if our gluteus medius is weak, then we develop a hip drop, functional short leg, and pelvic list or shift.

Primary muscles trained: Gluteals, hamstrings, spinal erectors, multifidus, transverses abdominals. (This exercise focuses on co-activation of the front and rear of your torso.)

Goal: 60 seconds (30 seconds left and 30 seconds right leg). Perform once for each leg or use multiple sets to achieve goal (e.g., 3 reps for 10 seconds each side).

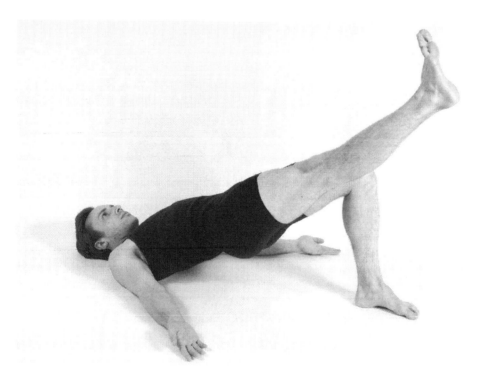

VIDEO 64: SINGLE LEG BACK BRIDGE

Back Bridge Using Two Legs

If a single-leg bridge is too challenging, start by keeping both feet planted. Forget about straightening the leg out until you build enough strength and endurance to accomplish the task. This is a good option for beginners.

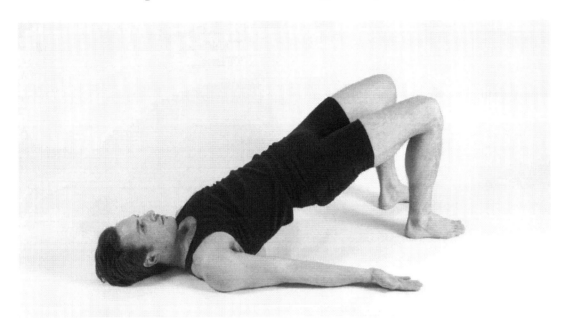

VIDEO 65: BACK BRIDGE USING TWO LEGS

Side Bridge (Advanced exercise, good for athletic people)

Lie on your side, lining up your thighs and torso in a straight line. Lean on your forearm, keeping the upper body supported. Then, abdominally brace and lift your torso upwards off the ground, balancing on just your ankles and forearm.

Primary muscles trained: abdominal obliques, quadratus lumborum, and gluteus medius.

Goal: 90 seconds. Perform once or use multiple sets to achieve goal (e.g., 6 reps for 15 seconds each).

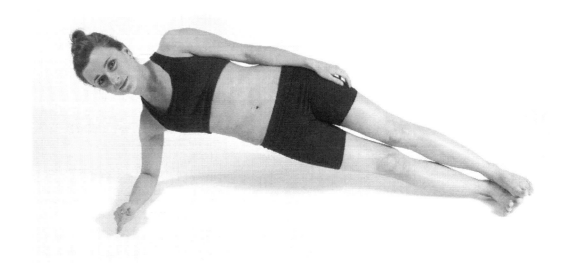

VIDEO 66: SIDE BRIDGE

Half-Side Bridge (Good for beginners)

If the side bridge is too challenging or you have shoulder or knee pain, then try this instead.

Simply bend the knees, keeping your hips and thighs in line with your torso. Lift your torso while balancing on your forearm and knees.

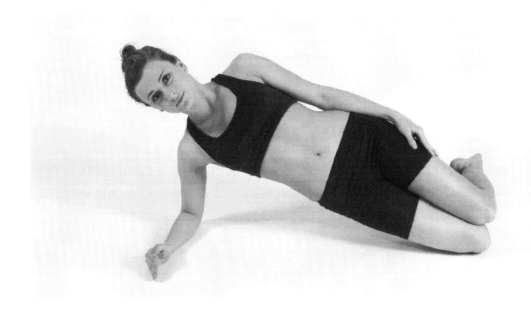

VIDEO 67: HALF-SIDE BRIDGE

Straight-Leg Torso Lift

If your shoulder can not support your upper body, you can accomplish strength to this region by performing this movement instead.

Simply lie on your side and stack your shoulders directly one on top of the other. Keep your hips, knees, and ankles all in one straight line with your spine and then lift your thighs off the ground.

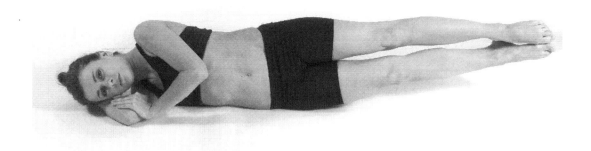

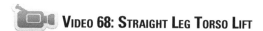 VIDEO 68: STRAIGHT LEG TORSO LIFT

Post Partum Abdominal Split

After giving birth women can develop a diastisis—a split in the abdominal wall where the two halves that are connected by a fibrous sheath literally split apart and create a crevus. Ab curls are an excellent way to help bridge the two halves together again. Remember to avoid the "loaf of bread" posture, as that will only make the split worse!

Ab Curls (Good for everyone.)

Perform an ab curl with hands tucked under your buttocks, and elbows flared out to the side and lifted upward. Keep one knee bent and the other straight with toes flexed upward. Pull your belly button inward and activate all abdominal muscles available, like you would with abdominal bracing, and curl upward until your shoulder blades lift off the floor. Try to avoid the "loaf of bread" posture—this is when you perform an abdominal curl up and create a protruding abdomen which looks like a freshly baked loaf of bread. The loaf posture creates excessive intra-abdominal pressure against pain sensitive structures in your back, elevates blood pressure, and means you are only engaging your outer most muscular wall—missing the benefits of engaging the deepest layers of the abdomen to help stabilize your spine.

Primary Muscles Trained: Rectus Abdominus, Transverus Abdominus

Goal: 60 seconds (30 seconds left; 30 seconds right). Perform once or use multiple sets to achieve goal (e.g., 10 seconds × 3 each side).

When the ab curl becomes too easy, try placing your hands on your forehead during the movement to create a more challenging exercise.

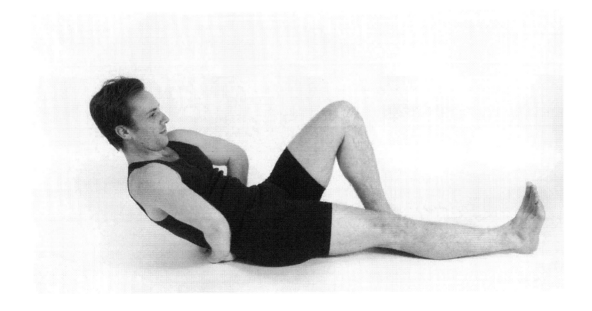

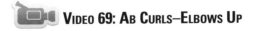 **VIDEO 69: AB CURLS—ELBOWS UP**

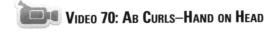 **VIDEO 70: AB CURLS—HAND ON HEAD**

Point and Reach (Good for everyone)

Get on all fours, lift one arm out in front of you, and lift the opposite leg straight out behind you. Reach both forwards and backwards at the same time as if you were being 'pulled' apart. Tighten the abdomen and hold the position.

This exercise is excellent because it utilizes co-activation of your front abdominals, lower back erectors, and hip extensors, keeping the spine safe with small spinal loads: about 25% on the upper back side and 25% on the lower back side with opposite arm and legs engaged. This way, we build endurance and co-activation without harming the lumbar spine.

Primary Muscles Trained: Erector Spinae, Multifidus, Abdominals, Glutes, Hamstrings, Scapular Stabilizers.

Goal: 2 minutes (1 minute per side). Perform for 15 seconds, switch arm and leg, and then repeat until goal is achieved. (Try touching your elbow and knee between reps and repeat for 15 second sets before switching sides.)

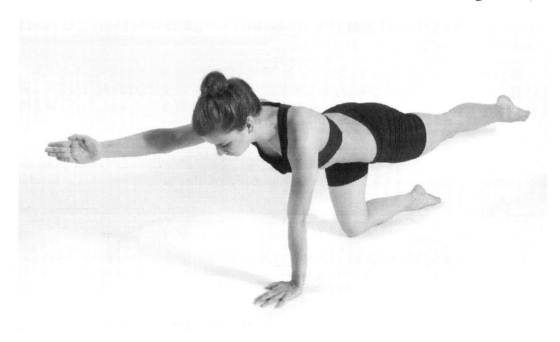

🎥 VIDEO 71: POINT AND REACH

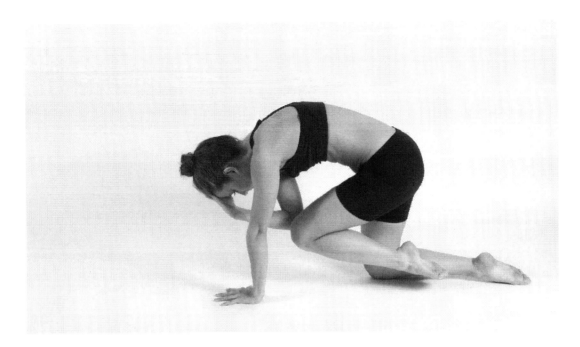

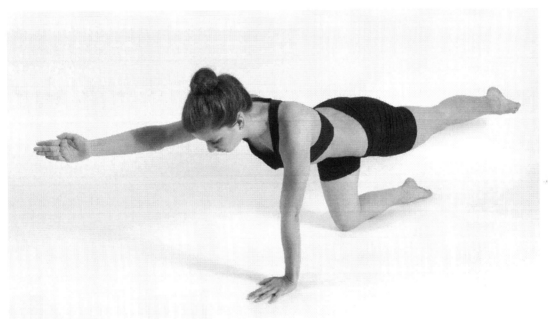

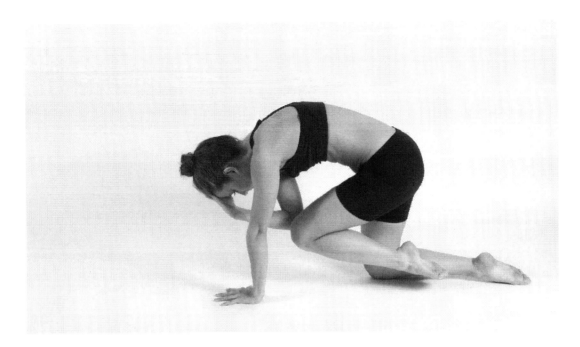 **VIDEO 72: POINT AND REACH—ELBOW KNEE**

Cat and Cow (Good for everyone)

Finish the program with a gentle cat/cow posture movement to leave your back lubricated.

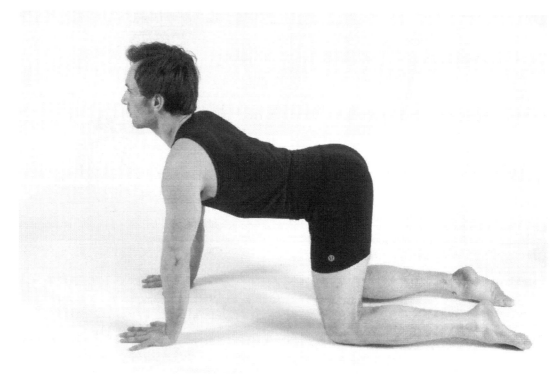

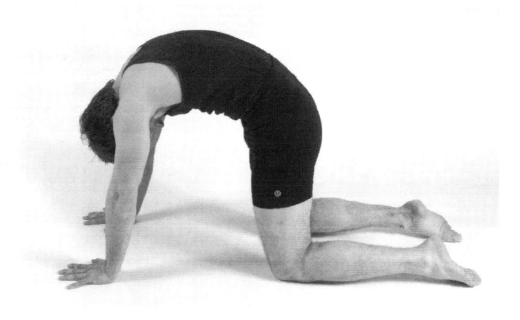

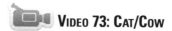

VIDEO 73: CAT/COW

Brace and Stand Up (Good for everyone)

While on all fours, find your neutral spine, engage your torso and abdominal muscles, and stand up.

Remember, the imbalance of endurance among the front, side, and lower back muscles remains long after lower back pain resolves. To prevent lower back trouble from reoccurring, maintain a regular schedule of the prescribed core routine—once a week is okay, but the more you do the routine, the more stable your back becomes. Experts say lower back exercises appear to be most beneficial when performed daily. It takes time, but your endurance will build and the routine will become easier to execute, especially because the core exercises have a specific sequence in which they are to be performed. They can be a part of your software update while you are building an anatomical corset. Perform each exercise one time or use multiple sets to achieve said goal time and execute both the left and right sides when appropriate. The time it will take to reach your goal depends on your physical condition, so don't get discouraged. It's not all about strength, it's about endurance, and building endurance takes time, just like someone training for a marathon. Finally, remember to perform the isometric exercises for your neck in order to avoid the possibility of straining it.

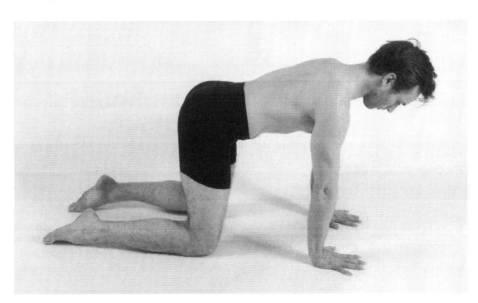

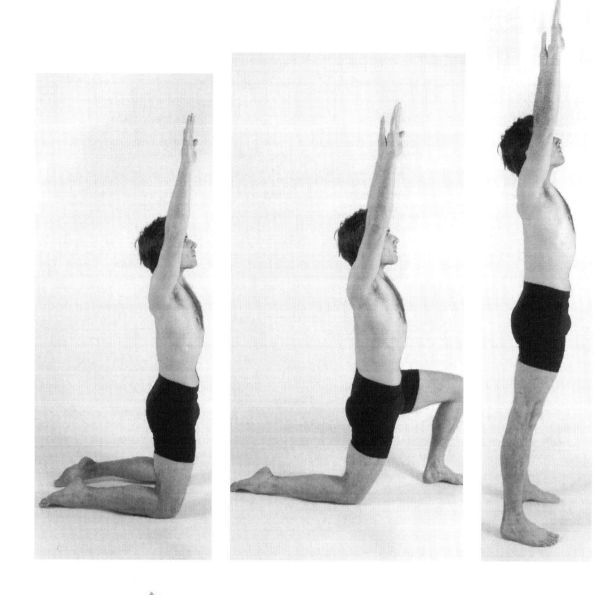

🎥 VIDEO 2: KNEELING TO STANDING ABDOMINAL BRACING

If necessary, use a chair to hold onto while trying to kneel, lunge, and eventually stand. All the while, keep your abdominal muscles engaged and strong.

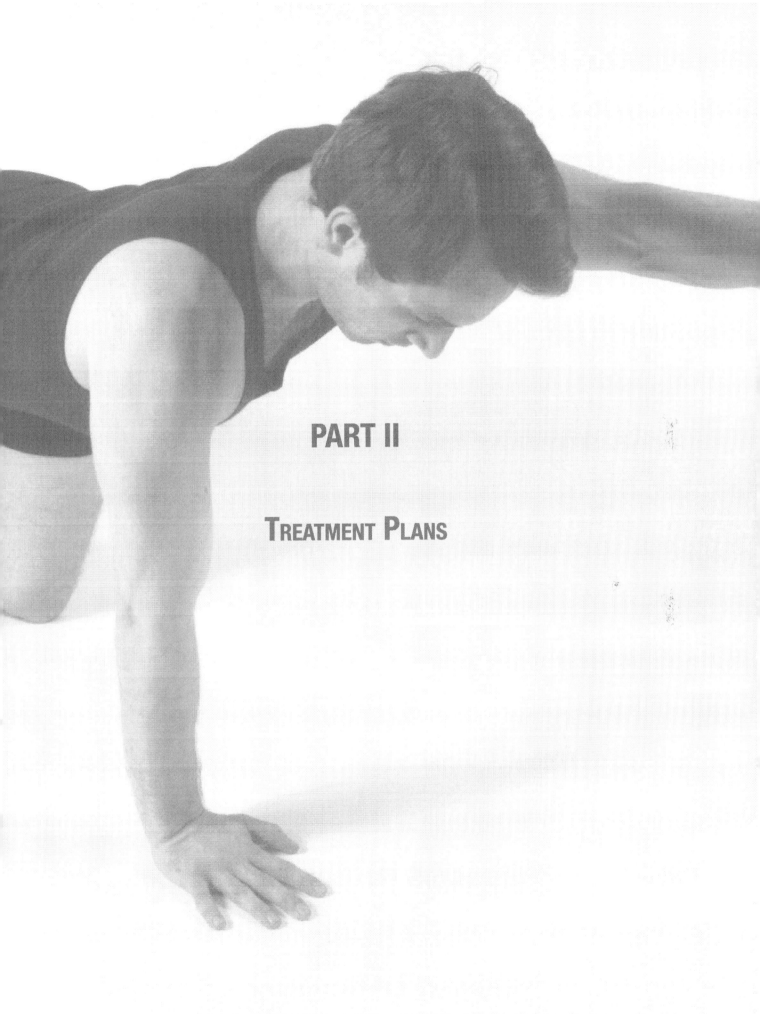

PART II

TREATMENT PLANS

4

On-The-Spot Self Care

"It is more important to know what sort of person has a disease than to know what sort of disease a person has."

—Hippocrates (460–377 B.C.)

LOWER BACK PAIN CAN BE DECEPTIVE, with symptoms that may resolve in just a few weeks, leading you to believe you are healed. However, thinking that the absence of pain means you're back to health is not just wrong, it can be dangerous. Symptoms are usually indicators of a deeper, darker problem that, when ignored, can become chronic and cause recurrent back attacks. While my goal is for you to avoid having to go straight to the doctor's office, I don't want you to avoid treatment all together. I want to help you treat yourself!

The biggest problem with going to a primary care doctor is that his or her advice may not be up to date. Many low back sufferers initially had a mechanical problem that was mismanaged by their physicians, unfortunately and I am certain that most of my colleagues would agree that primary care physicians are not experts on low back pain. They often send patients to a spinal expert, such as an orthopedic surgeon. Since only two to three percent of spinal injuries are surgical cases, however, he or she won't be very interested in the case once they determine surgery isn't required. Then, you're sent off to a physical therapist, recommended to you primarily on his or her proximity to your home or office, rather than expertise. So now you're back at square one, relying on the knowledge of yet another professional who may not be a spinal expert.

What follows is the most up-to-date, scientifically-proven, and peer-approved self-management techniques. This self-assessment, as well as being a self-treatment program, ensures that you're doing everything possible to avoid becoming a chronic pain sufferer.

Does Back Pain Ever Stop?

Twenty percent of lower back pain sufferers report additional episodes of back attacks for which they do not use medical services. This statistic means that most research reports on lower back pain treatments for health insurance benefits are limited in their insight. Researchers are actually only studying health services used in single instances of patients seeking treatment for back pain (known as "episodes of care"). Insurance companies need to understand that there is a range and variety of individual experiences with chronic back pain. In other words, most chronic lower back pain sufferers vary between episodes of pain and episodes of care. Many of these individuals report that they experience ongoing back pain that continues beyond their episodes of care and they use prescription drugs, medical services, and other health services only intermittently. This means that non-use of medical services does not equate to an individual being pain free.

Most people experience episodic recurrence of back pain, but most insurance carriers will deny medical coverage after one episode. This may be an indicator of why prescription drugs are used to treat back pain. It may seem as if people are having intermittent, recurring bouts of back problems, while in actuality, they are experiencing persistent pain in a continuous series of time periods but are not receiving additional medical care. Instead, they are taking prescription drugs to get them through until they seek care again.

How many times has a doctor heard a patient report having a bad back? Most patients receive varying diagnoses of their back problems over time from health care providers. These diverse diagnoses can potentially impair how insurance companies and medical researchers report, interpret, and decode back pain cases and can also yield broad, inconclusive representations of whether the back pain episode is acute, chronic, episodic, recurrent, or persistently continuous. The bottom line is that many patients report ongoing back pain that continues beyond their episodes of care and many with persistent back pain use prescription drugs and medical services only intermittently.

Self-Evaluation

The following is a quick guide to judging your back pain, along with advice on how to proceed. Read through the entire evaluation system and familiarize yourself with it so that if you find yourself in a back attack situation, you'll know how to proceed.

NOTE: THIS NEVER REPLACES THE PROPER ATTENTION BY YOUR SPINAL HEALTH CARE PROVIDER. WHEN IN DOUBT, SEE YOUR BACK DOCTOR.

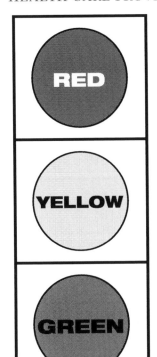

If you have any red lights, then immediately go see your doctor or go to the hospital

If you have any yellow lights, don't be alarmed, start my program and if after two weeks you are not significantly improved or your symptoms change or worsen, go see your doctor

Okay, you've evaluated yourself and you don't have anything seriously wrong that requires emergency care. Stay calm, stay active, start my program, and do not deviate unless your symptoms worsen.

Red Light: If you have lower back pain and have any of the below signs or symptoms, please go to your doctor or a local hospital.

A red light can potentially be indicative that your back pain may be a serious disease, which could cause death or paralysis.

- Age <20 or >55 years old
- Trauma related to pain (slip, fall, accident)
- Personal history of cancer
- Chest or middle back pain
- Night pain that wakes you up
- Fever, chills, night sweats, nausea, vomiting, diarrhea
- Steroid use
- Pain at rest (nothing mechanical makes it worse or better, it's just always there)
- Recent infection, now low back pain
- Saddle anesthesia: a complete numbness to your groin, like sitting on a horse
- Sphincter disturbance: inability to control bladder or bowel movements, including incontinence
- Motor weakness in the lower limbs, foot drop, tripping over foot, inability to walk on toes or heels, or inability to lift thigh to walk properly or do a single leg squat

 Yellow Light: Use caution. You don't have something seriously wrong yet, but be aware of your situation.

First Time Backache

- Very common
- Full recovery—may vary—but takes days or weeks to achieve
- Recurrence is possible—but doesn't mean re-injury
- Activity is helpful—bed rest is not!
- Hurting does not mean harm

Nerve pain, numbness, burning or tingling down one leg

- Don't be alarmed
- Pain down leg but not past your knee is better than pain down to your toes
- IF THE PAIN IN YOUR LEG STARTS TO CAUSE ANY RED LIGHT FLAGS, SUCH AS FOOT DROP OR GROIN NUMBNESS, THEN YOU SHOULD GO TO THE DOCTOR.
- Physician referral should be considered if you are not considerably better and have not returned to ordinary activities within 1–2 weeks.
- Usually takes 30–60 days to get rid of leg pain
- Full recovery is expected
- Recurrence is possible—but doesn't mean re-injury
- Some tests may be needed—MRI, x-ray, etc.
- Don't get down or withdraw from social interaction—go out with your friends
- Stay positive
- Active participation is essential
- Don't rely on someone fixing you…you need to fix yourself

 Green Light: You can take care of your back on your own.

You've evaluated yourself; you don't have anything seriously wrong that requires immediate emergency care. So, stay calm, stay active, and follow my advice daily.

Back pain can go away by itself, but don't get fooled. If you don't manage it properly, it will return and will probably be worse than before. It will probably take longer to improve, and may not ever fully resolve. If this is your first back attack and you follow my advice, chances are you will have a full recovery, never to have back pain again.

Immediate Self Care Techniques for Acute Pain and Recently Injured or Re-Injured Lower Back

1. **Use ice compresses** on your lower back for 15 minutes at a time (on for 15 minutes and off for 45 minutes) as much as possible for the first day, then 3–4 times every day for the next week. Don't keep ice on for longer than 15 minutes because your body will think its freezing, send more blood to the area, and cause it to heat up and become further inflamed. This does exactly the opposite of what you wanted to do in the first place. Always place a barrier between you and the ice pack (like a towel) to avoid ice burn.

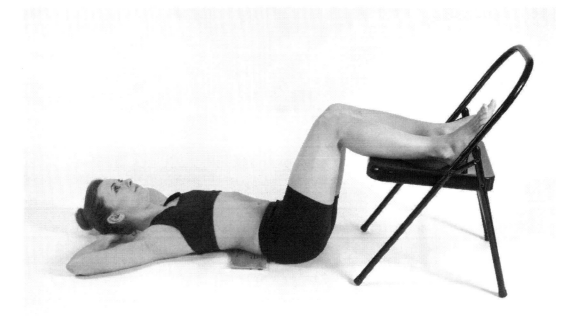

2. **Do not use heat.** This will cause further inflammation, worsen the pain, and probably make your low back pain linger.
3. **Try a lower back corset or belt**. This should provide relief by supporting your pelvis and allowing your muscles, which are probably in spasm, a chance to relax so they don't have to work so hard to stabilize your spine. This is fine for 72 hours, or, in a difficult case, 1–2 weeks at most. Like anything else with medicine, don't get hooked into using a brace all the time; our bodies need to heal with function, and the brace is like a crutch, in that it's there to help until you are healed.

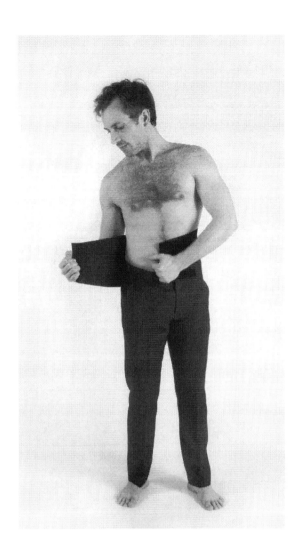

 VIDEO 74: LOWER BACK BELT

4. **Take over-the-counter NSAIDs** (non-steroidal anti-inflammatory medications like Ibuprofen or Naproxysodium) or other over-the-counter anti-inflammatories (ex. Advil, Motrin, Aleve). Call your primary doctor first and ask if over the counter NSAIDs are okay for you to take. If they are, use them for up to one week then discontinue, as stomach upset and bleeding ulcers are common side effects.

Do not take pain medicines or muscle relaxers. They have been proven to delay healing and prolong recovery with regards to lower back pain. Think about it—a muscle spasm is there to protect your spine from further injury. Why relax the muscles that are trying to help you and provide that protection? Back pain is very rarely the direct result of muscle trauma. Usually, the injury is to a ligament or nerve and the muscle spasms to help protect the integrity of your spine. A muscle relaxer removes that protection for the actual underlying cause of the pain, which is the reason why it's proven to delay healing and prolong recovery. If you feel you really need something to take the edge off, then by all means take the pain meds, but try to take them in the evening to help get a restful night's sleep.

5. **Stay comfortably active**. Walk around, go to work if possible, and avoid prolonged sitting, stooping, bending, or lifting. My suggestion for work is to stand up and perform the standing *Back in Action* exercises every hour to help prevent further pain and disability. These movements will promote healing. If your job is physically dangerous, then please obtain medical clearance.

6. **Avoid bed rest**. If you decide to stay home, research has proven that bed rest delays healing: for every day of bed rest it can take up to three additional days to heal your back. So, avoid being a couch potato and staying home in bed for days on end. It's simple math that if you take bed rest for three days it will result in nine extra days of recovery. We need your body to heal with mobility, otherwise it heals with sedentary properties that are not strong physiologically and will not be able to handle the stress of maintaining an upright posture (i.e., it makes your muscles weak). If you need to rest, then rest for small periods of time, say 30–60 minute intervals, and try these safe bed rest and sleeping postures (remember to keep the painful side up toward the ceiling if you lie on your side).

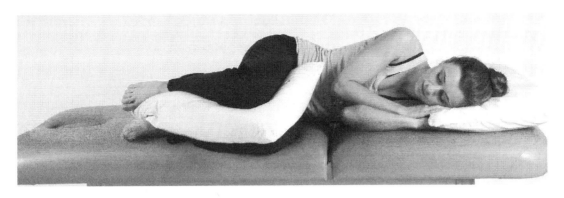

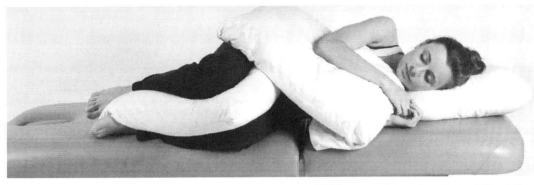

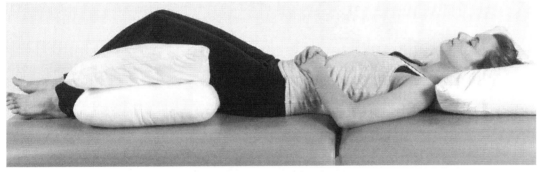

Sleeping on your stomach compresses the spine, shortens the muscles, and over arches the normal curvature. Avoid this posture at all costs. Whether you're in pain or not, it's a horrible sleeping position for the spine.

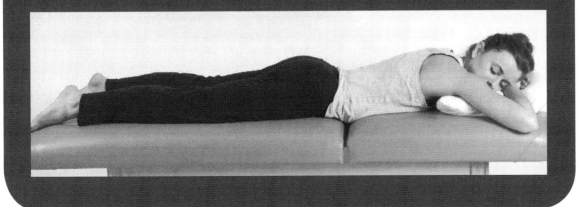

7. **Use abdominal bracing.** We discussed this earlier in great detail: if you are in acute pain—as a quick reference to help you stabilize your back—tighten all the muscles in your stomach as if someone is about to punch you in the gut. This will help you develop your own anatomical brace to support your injured back. Utilize this concept during any lifting task or transitional movements, such as rolling over in bed. Picture your core as a log, tighten your abs, and then roll over. If you do not tighten your core before rolling, the spine shears and causes pain.

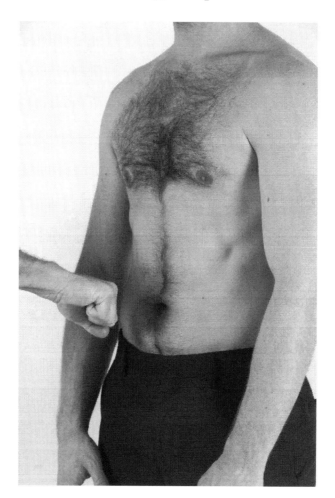

8. **Don't stretch your lower back**, especially if you just injured it! Avoid the temptation to stoop or bend forward, no matter how achy or stiff your back feels. The ache is a symptom of probable ligament sprains and disc tears; your muscles are simply overworking to protect your back. Stretching forward will only deactivate the lower back muscles, creating an environment of greater instability and the potential to further injure the tissues and cause more harm.

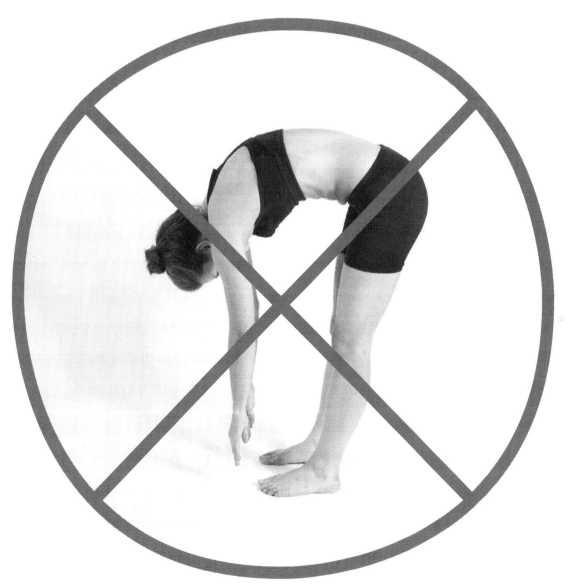

DON'T STRETCH YOUR LOWER BACK WHEN IT IS INJURED!

9. **Try arching your back**. When in doubt, especially when first injured, try arching backward slightly while standing as a first-course treatment. Then try to lie on your stomach and rest with your forehead resting on your arms. Physical therapists have built entire careers teaching patients to arch backward when they have back pain. The truth is, it's not always great to bend backward, as in the case of chronic lower back pain. But in an acute situation where you just injured or re-injured the spine, it's okay to try. Generally, if a disc is herniated or torn, it has a tendency to protrude backward towards the spinal canal. If you adopt a stretch in a forward posture, you essentially push the gel of the disc further into the spinal canal, worsening the disc protrusion. By bending backwards, you create a physical force that pulls the gel material of the disc back into the disc itself, taking the gel away from painful spinal structures. The bottom line is, if you injure your back, try arching backwards as a first line of defense and avoid the temptation to flex forward.

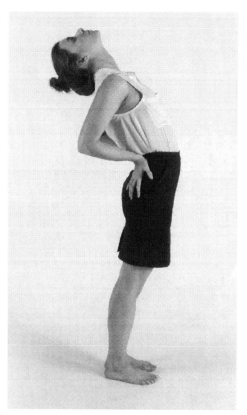

Try back arching, especially when first injured.

I'm Crooked and I Can't Stand Up

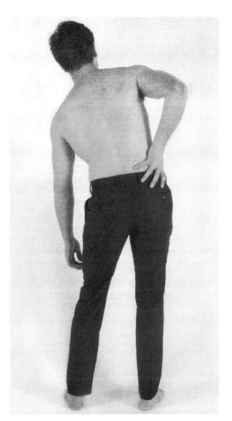

Antalgia—shifting to one side—is a normal response to back pain (right)

When you hurt your back, sometimes the spine shifts to one side or the other to alleviate pressure and pain. This is called antalgia, and it's a normal response to back pain and is how the body works to alleviate pain. Most people think they have a back spasm, but what they don't realize is that they probably injured their discs. You do not need sciatica (pain caused by general compression or irritation of one of five spinal nerve roots of each sciatic nerve) to have a disc injury. Try the standing pelvic shift movements (next) to realign your spine. It's normal to have a slight increase in discomfort while practicing these moves until your pelvis glides into normal alignment.

Standing Pelvic Shift

Simply look in a full length mirror to determine which direction your pelvis has shifted, then, using the below movements, try to glide your pelvis back into alignment. This will help alleviate the lower back discomfort and take the unequal weight pressure off the disc, which will allow it to heal.

Simply lean your forearm against a wall and use your other arm to gently push your pelvis toward the wall in an effort to align your spine. Hold for 10 seconds.

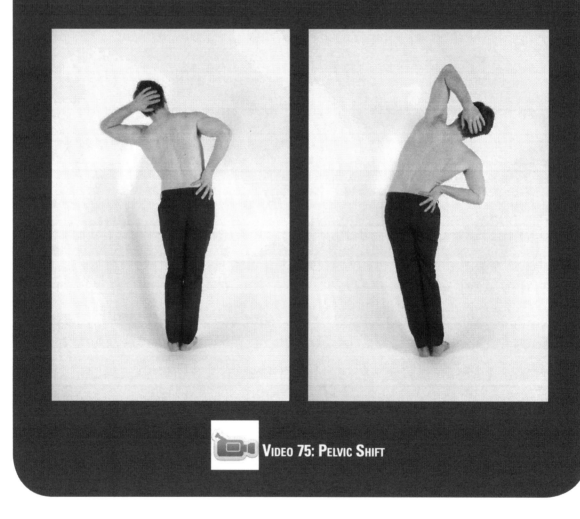

VIDEO 75: PELVIC SHIFT

Sciatica

If you have pain, numbness, or burning in your buttock, thigh, back of thigh, calf, or down into your foot, you probably have a nerve irritation called sciatica, an inflammation or compression to a tree-trunk nerve from being hit by a bone, disc, ligament, or some other space-occupying lesion. A pinch at your spine is like a short in an electrical wire that sends mixed signals down your entire leg into your foot.

When your sciatic nerve is compressed, it causes inflammation. This inflammation causes a cascade of irritants, which yield pain. When the inflammation calms down, as it does with the use of ice or anti-inflammatories, pain disappears and people think they are better. Unfortunately, this is not the case. The byproduct of inflammation is scar tissue, which is called fibrinogen. This scarred tissue is laid down over the path of inflammation and, in the case of sciatica, maybe the entire leg. Most people think scar tissue is only formed by a cut on your skin that heals with a scab, but scar tissue can form anywhere in the body. It can form in women who had ovarian cysts or uterine fibroids. It forms in and around muscles that were previously injured, like torn hamstrings, rotator cuffs, and pulled calf muscles.

Think of scarred tissue as you would a fatty marbleized steak. Instead of a red, lean piece of beef, you have a ropey, non-tender, fatty piece of meat! Sorry for the analogy, but it's pretty accurate. Remember, scar tissue is non-elastic. It rips and tears very easily. When this happens, it causes a temporary inflammation that builds up more scar tissue adhesions when it heals again. Thus, it's a cycle of injury, inflammation, and scar tissue. As this cycle continues, scar tissue begins to form a spider web of adhesions, which stick together and attach themselves to surrounding structures, and in this case, to your sciatic nerve. Now, every time you take a step, the scar tissue tugs at your sciatic nerve, physically pulling on it and creating nerve irritation. Remember, this pull can be at the spinal canal where the nerve originates, or further down the leg, like deep in the buttocks, hamstring, calf, or foot.

To break this cycle, we need to break up the scar tissue and prevent it from playing tug-of-war on your sciatic nerve. This is how we do it—flossing. Think of sciatic flossing the same way you glide floss between your teeth, breaking up debris so it doesn't cause plaque. Only, instead of using floss, you're using your sciatic nerve, gently gliding it back and forth from your lower back, down your leg to your toes, and then back up again to your spine. The idea is to keep gliding your nerve to essentially free it from obstruction. Otherwise, the scar tissue will continue to glue itself to your nerve and cause pain.

Perform these movements several times a day until your sciatic pain is relieved. Initially, trying to floss your sciatic nerve may increase or exacerbate symptoms, but don't be discouraged. Just apply ice to three places: (1) the lower back, (2) buttock, and (3) back of the knee afterwards for 5 minutes each. This ensures that you cool down the sciatic nerve at the three most vulnerable locations. If after one to two weeks these spinal movements do not cure or lessen the sciatic pain, then please see your doctor.

Hold each posture for 5 seconds. Make the movements as smooth as possible and try not to jerk your body into position. Expect an increase in symptoms initially, but then they should subside. If your symptoms worsen, then by all means, stop the movements immediately and go see your doctor.

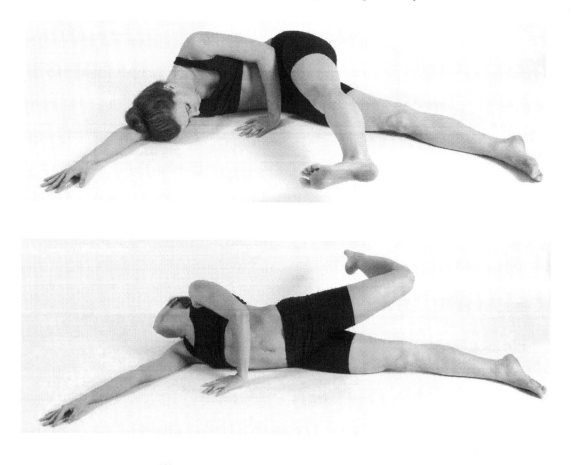

VIDEO 76A: LYING SCIATICA FLOSSING

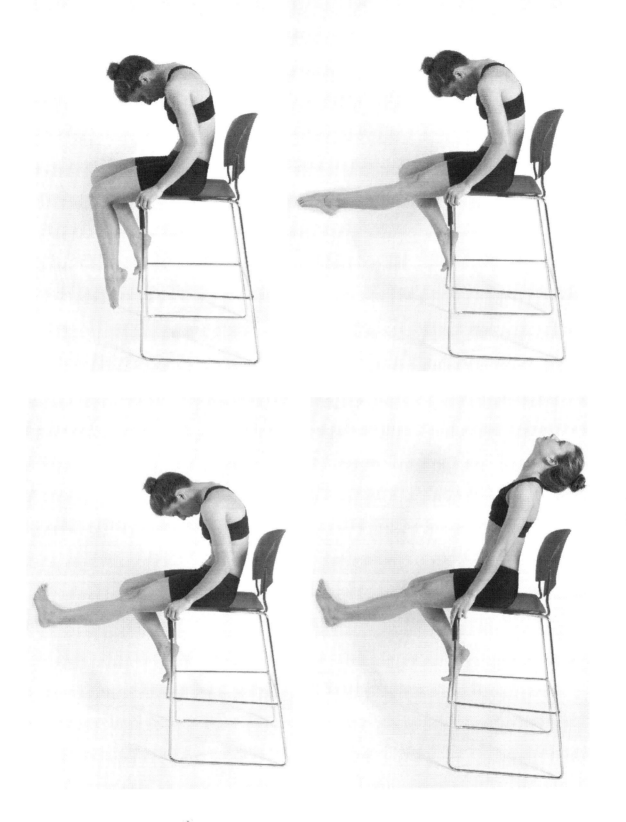

VIDEO 76B: SEATED SCIATICA FLOSSING

Future Predictors of Low Back Pain

Who will suffer and who will not? That is the question. It turns out the most accurate and clinically tested, foolproof prediction of future back pain is your personal history. The longer it has been since your last back attack, the lower your chance for a reoccurrence. The shorter the time from your last attack, the greater the chance for further ongoing back pain. In other words, the likelihood of further back attacks becomes diminished with the time since your last attack.

Time Since Last Attack	Likelihood of future back pain during next 12 months
One Week	>75%
About 1 Month	>60%
Between 1-12 Months	>50%
Between 1-5 Years	>40%
More than 5 years	>30%

All data are based on known medical data (Hestbaek et al. 2003; Bronfrot et al. 2008). When most acute episodes of low back pain improve, patients stop consulting doctors and return to their normal lives. However, only a minority fully recover. Here's the low down:

The Good

Those of you who experience an acute episode of low back pain will get better, pain-wise, to a point where you don't feel the need to consult a doctor and you can return to your normal lives in about 6 weeks on average.

Improvements on average (what you can expect):

- Week 1 = 25% improvement
- Weeks 2–3 = 50% improvement
- Weeks 4–5 = 75% improvement
- Weeks 6+ = 90–100% improvement

The Bad

Despite the fact that your pain levels have improved, functional activities of daily living lag behind. History tells us that 70% of first time back sufferers continue to have residual, nagging problems (stiffness, difficulty with bending, stooping, and lifting, etc.) during the next year.

The Ugly

Here's the ugly: only a minority of you will feel fully recovered in the sense of being completely symptom free. On average, 12 months after an acute episode of lower back pain, only 25% of you will be completely symptom free. Over 75% of us learn, adapt, self-manage, and seek help from others to alleviate our ongoing aches and pains.

These figures seem to be consistent in the clinical series of medical research over the past 40 years. However, those predictions are based on the past experiences of low-back-pain sufferers who appear to have been mismanaged. So much has changed over that period, which is partly why I wrote this book: to bring you to the 21st century of healthcare for lower back pain. So, don't get discouraged, start today, and let's change history together.

Disability and Low Back Pain

How long do people who suffer with lower back pain stay out of work? According to data collected over the last 25 years, on average, during a back attack episode:

- 40% return to work within 1 week
- 70% return to work within 2 weeks
- 80% return to work within 1 month
- 90% return to work within 3–6 months
- 10% never return to work.

The longer a patient is off from work due to back pain, the lower the chance they will return to work at all. When someone does not show up to work because of back pain, there's a 10% chance they'll still be off from work one year later.

If you don't return to work within the following time frames, the coinciding percentages below may apply:

- 4–6 weeks = 20% chance of long term disability
- 6 months = 50% chance of long term disability
- 1+ years = it's unlikely you will ever work again.

The further you slide down this slippery slope, the harder it is for you to climb back up. Despite your physical condition or any health care you receive, the passage of time itself changes the whole situation. Clinical management should be simple symptomatic relief, patients should be provided tips and exercise advice to support recovery, and return to ordinary activities as early as possible. When this is not done (or when it is done incorrectly) low back pain endures and disaster sets in physically, emotionally, and financially. All of a sudden, what started as an ordinary backache has become a major source of suffering and disability. People become trapped in a vicious circle of low back pain, disability, and failed treatments. The longer someone is in pain, the less likely it is that rehabilitation will succeed. These chronic pain sufferers are a small subgroup of people, a 10–15% minority, but they have a disproportionate impact on health care use and social costs. They develop emotional and behavioral problems that are out of proportion with their physical problems.

Chronic pain is basically pain that continues to be present as though the patient still has an acute problem. The main difference is the impact the pain has on someone's life. What we want to look for in these cases are factors that delay recovery in the acute stage of someone's pain, as compared to what most doctors do now, which is to look for factors that cause chronic pain. If you want to prevent lower back pain from becoming chronic, treat it early, treat it correctly, and treat it simply!

Disability is a disaster in terms of its economic impact on the patient who is out of work, their employability, the need for their retraining or replacement, escalating health care costs, financial support from society, and possible adversarial legal proceedings. The principle of prevention is better than the cure. It's much easier to prevent a lower back attack from becoming chronic than it is to reverse the problem once it becomes intractable pain.

Back Belts

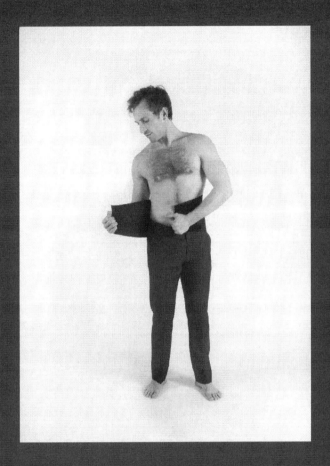

 VIDEO 77: LOWER BACK BELT

In the case of an acute injury, you may do well to use a back belt to help you function and allow you to practice your own abdominal bracing. For acute low back pain during a back attack, a low back corset belt—an elastic belt with crossed bands and metal reinforcement in the back—is effective in reducing low back pain and helping heal the injury.

Back Belts (continued)

Why? Because back belts keep the patient functional; that is, they can sit, stand, and bend with less strain on the spine, allowing the soft tissues (discs, joints, ligaments, and muscles) to relax so they can heal. It also limits forward bending (flexion), which we know is horrible for the lower back. Finally, it controls posture and educates body alignment to keep the spine in a neutral and slightly extended posture. This ensures a locking mechanism for the spinal joints and trains the muscles for adaptation of this posture.

If you have a sedentary job (i.e., you mostly sit all day), then wear the brace the second half of the day when your muscles are most fatigued until adequate healing has taken place. Again, use the belt no longer than a one- to two-week period, as spinal deconditioning atrophy and fatty infiltration penetrate the very muscles you need to stabilize your spine.

Here's the skinny on back belts for you employers out there—evidence suggests that uninjured workers who wear back support belts have a higher risk of injury and higher cost of treatment than those who injure their backs not wearing a belt.

Apparently, wearing a back belt tricks you into thinking you can lift more than you should. It creates faulty muscle patterns, which grossly change lifting techniques, so that when the belt is off, you lift something awkwardly and injure your spine because your body was used to the added support. Therefore, back belts do not prevent injuries among uninjured workers. Back belts also raise intra-abdominal pressure (like coughing, sneezing, or laughing), which increases lower back compression. Bottom line is, if your back doesn't hurt, then do not wear a belt because it makes you more prone to injury.

Note: Wearing the belt for 1–2 weeks while inflamed is fine, but wearing a belt longer than that can have the reverse effect and worsen your back via a deconditioning process. You can, however, wear the belt to work for an additional 2–4 weeks following an acute back attack if you have an occupation that requires bending, stooping, twisting, or lifting.

Worker's Compensation: The Blame Game

Who's to blame for your lower back pain? We already know that lower back attacks are spontaneous, unpredictable, and have no clear association with overexertion. However, people need something or someone to blame...work, sports, pregnancy, child birth, housework, yard work, gardening, kids, stress, posture tension, arthritis...should I keep going? Many people give more than one answer, and obviously the factors people blame vary at different stages of their lives.

In Canada, the Official Back Institute conducted a study of 8,000 people with lower back pain. What they found may surprise you. They reported that, of those patients who were responsible for their own health expenses, 66% said that they had no idea what caused their lower back pain.

In contrast, of those people who were not responsible for their own health care expenses, 90% blamed some kind of work event. Whether their job required light or heavy exertion made little difference. They lifted something, bent forward, or maybe sat too long. We all get low back pain. There is no one or nothing to blame unless you actually fell from a ledge or were struck by a brick. The truth is that we have very little information about what causes or even triggers lower back pain.

5

FITNESS AND BACK PAIN

"The greatest discovery of any generation is that human beings can alter their lives by altering the attitudes of their minds."

—ALBERT SCHWEITZER

I HAVE ALWAYS BELIEVED in the philosophy of "do as I do" as opposed to the old philosophy of "do as I say, not as I do." I recall a visit to the cardiologist in 1985 with my father who was suffering from heart disease. Outside of the office, there was the doctor in his lab coat, overweight, and smoking a cigarette. When we approached, my father said, "You told me smoking was bad for my heart." The doctor looked at my father, whom he already knew, and said exactly that old adage. I'll never forget it: "Abe, don't do as I do, do as I say." It was that exact moment that my philosophy of "do as I do" became the way I led my life.

I want to help all athletes and exercise enthusiasts stay active and continue to train even while healing an injury. Since knowledge is power, the more you understand about the mechanics of exercise and how it affects your spine, the better athlete you become. You cannot just spin, swim, and run. You have to stretch, engage your core, and self-manage to prevent injuries.

"No Pain, No Gain." This old adage is crap! If you perform a movement and it hurts your back, don't do it. The presence of pain prevents the development of healthy movement patterns because there is an adaptation of many muscle groups that activate in compensation for injured tissues. Instead, focus on the *Back in Action* and spine strengthening exercises that I outlined previously before you start engaging in sports, leisure activities, etc. This will help to prepare your spine for action and hopefully normalize mobility. However, if you continue to partake in sports while in pain, you will ingrain faulty movement patterns into your nervous system. Then, even when you are free of pain, you are set up to fail and reinjure your back while performing a normal activity of daily living.

Fit individuals injure their spines less frequently than unfit individuals. But, when they do injure their spines it is usually more severe, as they tend to challenge their spines by lifting more weights or taking greater risks with exercise than an unfit person does. Additionally, while unfit people tend to complain more about their minor aches and pains, many athletes will continue to compete despite their injury, often compounding the damage. The take-home message from all of this—do everything in moderation, regardless of your level of fitness!

When your back hurts or you are recovering from an episodic back attack, don't become inactive. Keeping aerobically fit will flush your injured back with oxygenated blood and nutrients to help heal your spine. By being aerobic, you elevate the oxygen supply to your blood stream, which then supplies this oxygen to all of your body parts. Your bloodstream carries all the additional healthy stuff that heals injured tissues and lubricates joints. Therefore, exercise can essentially act as anti-aging. So, here are my recommendations:

- If you are inactive, then get off your butt and start walking for about ten minutes a day.
- If you're mildly active (you participate in some type of exercise) then build up to being active for 30 minutes three times a week.
- If you are moderately active (you exercise regularly) then I encourage you to continue exercising; don't stop just because your back hurts. Instead, modify the kinds of exercise you do: walk instead of run, bike leisurely instead of taking a spin class, swim instead of using an elliptical trainer, and perform core exercises instead of weight training. However, you can continue to weight train, only focus on the upper body while leaving the lower body alone.

Here's a sample program for active folks and athletes:
- Go through the AM routine on page 48 to warm up (2 minutes).
- Perform aerobic activity for 30–40 minutes: use an elliptical trainer or treadmill, ride a bike, or take a brisk walk (30–40 minutes).
- Perform the core routine on page 134 (8 minutes).
- Train the upper body with weights if desired (every other day to rest muscles): vary the muscle groups of your upper body to prevent over-use injury, such as one day performing chest and arm exercises while the next day performing upper back and shoulder exercises. You get the picture.
- Stretch as prescribed on page 113 (5 minutes).

Being an athlete is not easy. Don't slow down: keep comfortably active until you are "Back in Action."

How to Train Your Core While Being Aerobic

When breathing heavily, our body struggles to activate the abdominals. This is an indicator of compromised spine stability. Whether you are an athlete or simply trying to stay in shape, you need to train your body to maintain an abdominal brace independent of labored breathing. Below is an excellent way to challenge your body to do so in order to prevent back pain while training to become aerobically fit.

Most athletes, when injured, say their knees are given a rehab program based purely on strength, power, range of motion, and flexibility. When undergoing rehab, rarely is any attention paid to a base foundation of spine strength during aerobic activity. This is a general recipe for lower back pain in athletes. Try the following 30-minute routine and watch how your core strength improves when you engage in sports again.

Sample 45-Minute Cardio Routine

- Run, bike, walk, elliptically train, whatever—just get yourself to a level of labored breathing (10 minutes).
- Immediately stop and perform the following exercises every 5 minutes during a cardio routine, such as:

> Side bridges left: 30 seconds
> Cardio: 5 minutes
> Side bridges right: 30 seconds
> Cardio: 5 minutes
> Ab curl, left leg straight: 30 seconds
> Cardio: 5 minutes
> Ab curl, right leg straight: 30 seconds
> Cardio: 5 minutes
> Plank: 30 seconds
> Cardio: 5 minutes
> Point and reach: 30 seconds left/right
> Cardio: 5 minutes
> Point and reach: 30 seconds left/right
> Cardio: 5 minutes

If or when this routine becomes too easy, increase the time of the core exercises or increase the intensity of the cardio workout to mimic the intensity of your sport.

Running and Low Back Pain

As a general rule of thumb, running doesn't cause low back pain. However, when a runner experiences back pain, it's usually for mechanical reasons. By that I mean pain from running is usually from mechanical compression of the facet joints of the spine combined with muscle tightness in the hips. The quadratus lumborum, TFL (tensor fasciae lata), IT band, piriformis, hamstrings, and hip flexors are generally to blame. This is particularly true with road running because of the banks on the roads where one side is elevated and the other depressed. If you run the same course in one direction constantly, you are setting your pelvis up for failure.

If you correct the mechanics via stretching after running and performing movement prep exercises prior to your runs, the back pain should disappear. I have had the great privilege to treat some of the world's greatest and fastest distance runners. If you want a taste of running greatness, check out my website www.dukechironyc.com. These athletes don't see me because there is necessarily something wrong or painful related to their backs, but seek advice to "tune" their bodies and help prepare for a race. They see me to optimize performance and prevent injury from the common effects of constant running, such as tight IT bands, pulling on the knee caps, shortening of stride due to muscle tightness in specific regions of the hips, or pelvic unleveling. Under normal conditions, the femur heads and tops of the pelvis should be exactly parallel to the surface. If one side is higher than the other, it can cause a shearing force in the hips, which can irritate one or several gluteal muscles.

I do anything I can to help athletes' bodies savor a feeling of effortless running; a running economy if you will. I try to help make their running journey easier with less pull and strain to create a more fluid movement. Essentially, I am the artist and they are my canvas. These runners usually see me for a pre-race tune up to help optimize performance. From my experiences with world-class runners, I have developed a routine for distance athletes and have discovered similar traits among all runners. My recommendations are similar for you. You don't have to be an Olympic athlete to be treated like one.

Perform the essential five stretches described on page 113 after a run to alleviate potential stressors placed on the lower back. However, never stretch before running. Remember, stretching deactivates muscles and you do not want to weaken the muscles of your legs prior to taking it out to the streets.

Instead, before a run perform some of the Standing Routine movements (see page 49) such as swimmer, backstroke, and golf twists. These limber your mid back while the pelvic twists, hip gyros and leg swings prepare your lower body.

Besides what I have already described to battle back pain, below are some recommendations specific for runners. Immediately after a run, perform the following routine.

Facet Decompression Stretch

This is the only place in this book you'll find this type of stretch. Perform immediately after any run. While standing, fold your hands behind your head and neck and, like a butterfly, open your elbows and breathe inward. Then, while breathing out, fold your elbows together, trying to press them together while you flex your head. Next, like a butterfly flapping its wings, open your elbows again whilst breathing in, and breathe out bringing your elbows together. Flex forward, further rolling your spine until you are almost placing your head between your knees. It usually takes 4–5 movements to get there, about 30 seconds or so.

This movement is designed to open your facet joints immediately after a run, during which they usually compress together, irritating the sensitive nerve endings of the joint capsules.

After decompressing the facet joints, perform the essential five stretches: (1) piriformis, (2) hip flexor, (3) standing flank, (4) hamstring, and (5) spinal erector. Then add one additional stretch—the three-way calf stretch.

Three-Way Calf Stretch

Tight calves wreak havoc on posture. When short and tight, they have a tendency to tilt the pelvis forward, creating an exaggerated swayback posture similar to the one that occurs when wearing high-heels. Combine this with the

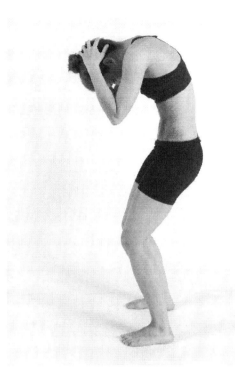
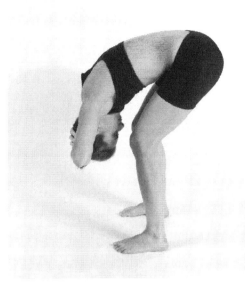

📹 **Video 78: Facet Decompression Stretch**

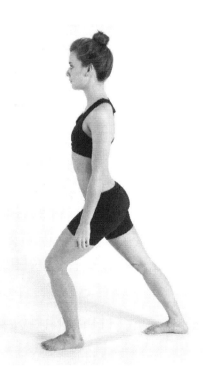
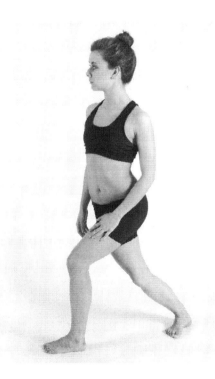

📹 **Video 79: Three-way Calf Stretch**

usual injuries associated with tight calves—like shin splints, stress fractures, foot and ankle tendonitis, and plantar fasciitis issues—and you can see why it becomes essential to stretch this area after running. Here are a few stretches you can do to avoid tight calves:

1. **Basic calf stretch**: Simply press your arms into a wall and lunge backwards, keeping your back leg straight and pressing your heel towards the ground. You should feel this stretch behind the knee where the calf muscles and hamstrings crisscross.

2. **Soleus stretch**: From the same position as the basic calf stretch, gently flex your back knee, again making sure to keep your heel on the ground. You should feel this stretch in the Achilles area.

3. **Tibialis posterior**: This is part of the posterior compartment and is responsible for shin, ankle, and foot-related problems. Form the same position as above and gently turn your back foot inward, then bend your knee again. You should feel the stretch on the inner part of the ankle.

4. Perform the following core routine:

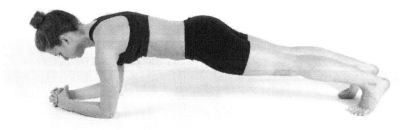

Front plank: 90 seconds

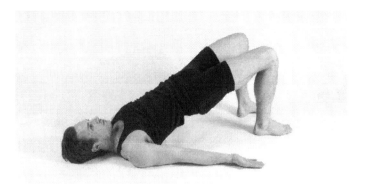

Back bridge: 60 seconds

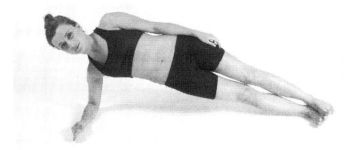

Side bridges: 180 seconds (90 seconds on each side)

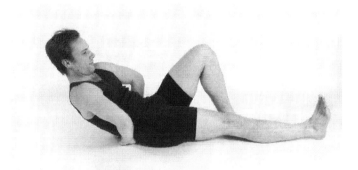

Ab curls: 60 seconds (30 seconds on each side)

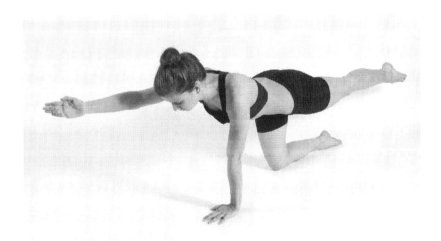

Point & reach: 120 seconds (60 seconds on each side)

If pressed for time, then just perform single-leg bridges for 60 seconds (30 seconds on each side)

5. **Single-leg bridges**: These will engage your glute medius, spinal erectors, and transverse abdominus, as well as build strength in them following the fatigue associated with an endurance run. It's a great way to train your body to avoid back pain by preventing hip drop to the pelvis and all the problems associated with it.

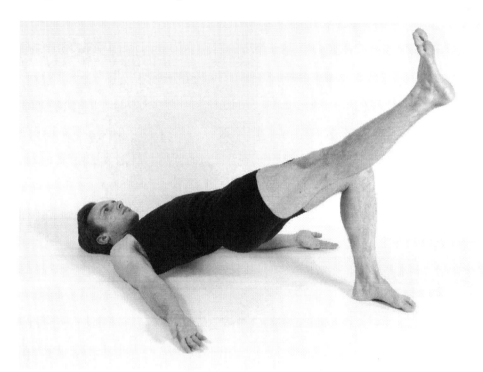

6. **Foam roller**: Use a foam roller that is 6 inches in diameter to knead out knots in your muscles. Doing this is an excellent way to knead out adhesions to the iliotibial band on the outer thigh and the piriformis deep in the glutes. Take a foam roller, place it on the floor, lie sideways with your hip on the roller, and with your upper body strength, simply roll up and down your thigh. While kneading out the tissue, you will probably find numerous hot spots that are very tender to pressure. When you do, stop the roller, bend your knees, and then roll some more, bending and straightening your knees throughout. The bending and straightening of the knees glides the hamstrings and quadriceps from under the IT band, releasing unwanted fibrous adhesions that build up from the microtrauma associated with running. Next, sit on the roller, cross one ankle over the opposite knee, and roll the buttocks. This movement will target the piriformis area.

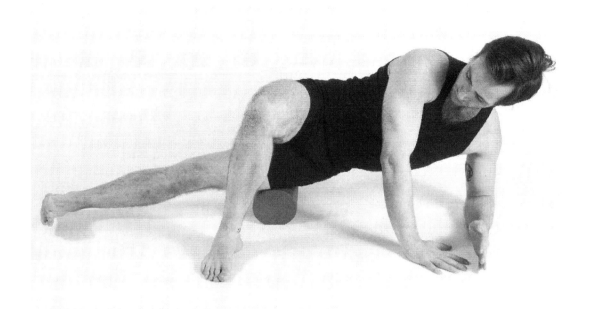

VIDEO 80: FOAM ROLLER FOR IT BAND

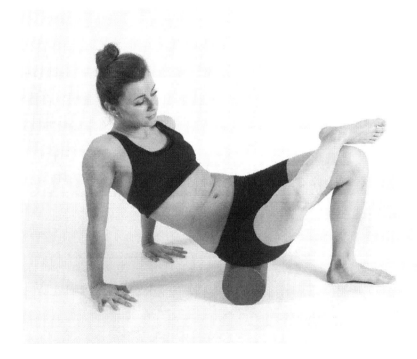

VIDEO 81: FOAM ROLLER FOR PIRIFORMIS

Yoga and the Back

Let me preface this section by saying I am a fan of yoga and practice myself. However, I am not a fan of large classes and of all the postures, as there are many postures which are unfortunately harmful to the spine. So, what comes to mind when you think of yoga? Well, if you think of a man or woman in seemingly impossible poses, then you may have an inkling of what yoga is. Yoga is an ancient Indian body of knowledge that dates back more than 5,000 years. The word "yoga" came from the Sanskrit word "yuj," which means to unite or integrate. Ancient yogis had a belief that in order for a man to be in harmony with his environment, he had to integrate the body, mind, and spirit. This is done though exercise, breathing, and meditation—the three main yoga structures. Sounds nice, doesn't it? Meditation, relaxation, breathing, one with nature… But why do so many yoga practitioners come to me with back problems?

I blame it on the large corporate studios competing with each other by trying to be unique and offering yoga as a way to break a sweat and lose weight. They have ruined yoga by trying to make it a workout and attempting to brand the practice of yoga as a merely physical endeavor instead of the spiritual practice it actually is. One of the biggest culprits of this misunderstanding may be "power yoga," a type of yoga in which instructors rush students through complicated poses, walking around the studio and literally pushing people into a pose when they are having difficulty getting themselves into a posture. They do not consider that the person may well have a structural deficit that prohibits them from getting into that pose.

I once had a patient who took a gym yoga class regularly. One day, a different instructor than usual showed up. When my patient couldn't get into a certain pose, the instructor came over and pushed her into it. The woman immediately felt severe spinal pain. The instructor told her such pain was part of yoga, that it was teaching her body to adapt to the pose, and that her spine should allow this motion. Anyway, this woman found her way to my office where we took x-rays of her spine and found she had a condition known as spondylolisthesis, where the vertebrae in the lower back slip forward. She had never had a problem with it before. She explained to me that yoga really felt fine as long as she limited her range of motion. However, since the new instructor had pushed her spine into a backwards arch and overexerted her natural ability to extend her spine, she was in a lot of pain.

I had another patient who practiced yoga seven times a week for two hours a day. She came to my office with moderate back pain that yoga didn't resolve. She said that, initially, the yoga had helped with the pain, but it had eventually stopped working. I switched her from yoga to core strength training. I kept her spine safe and stable while strengthening her core. Six weeks later, all of her back pain had been resolved. The yoga had created hypermobility (overstretching) in her joints in the spine so that she required stabilization exercises to alleviate her pain.

The moral of these stories: personal trainers, yoga instructors, coaches, therapists, and so on do not have x-ray vision. If you feel uncomfortable with a certain posture, then that posture is probably not good for you. This is why I suggest staying away from large yoga classes if you have back pain.

Yoga is seen by many as a useful way to strengthen your core muscles, including your back. This is incorrect. If you have already had back attacks, you should avoid doing yoga, especially without proper supervision.

Even though I generally do not recommend yoga for anyone with lower back pain, it may be helpful, but only if you avoid poses that hyperflex (round the lower back while bending forward) the spine or place an overexertion of extension (arching backwards, creating a sway back) on the spine. I take x-rays, perform examinations, look at anatomy, and so on to make my determinations. So, when I do recommend it, I tailor all movements for my patient's spine and the instructors that I recommend understand that my patients must follow my advice during class. There are too many variables involved with yoga that can potentially harm the back. However, if you do have lower back pain and you're determined to take a yoga class, you must tell the teacher about your lower back pain before starting the class. Be careful with health club yoga classes—they are generally meant for the masses and not tailored toward individuals with back pain. I encourage you to find a yoga studio in your town where the instructor has a minimum of 200 hours (and preferably more) of yoga instruction and to communicate with your doctor. A certified yoga instructor will listen to you and alter poses based on your comfort level. He or she will also recommend the use of props to help you achieve poses without straining your back. Once in the class, keep to the basics. Meditate, relax, and learn to breathe deeply.

Spine Safe Yoga Poses

There are several exercises we've talked about in the Back in Action plan that are similar to yoga poses. Below are just a few of some common yoga poses that are beneficial to the back. Though there are more, these are most similar to the "Back in Action" routine movements.

Cat and Cow

Begin on all fours with your back parallel to the floor. While breathing out, curl your body into a U-shape, bringing your tailbone and head up, then breathe in while rounding your back and bringing your head down toward your chest. This pose is a good stretch to create movement and flexibility in your back.

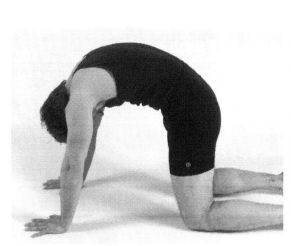 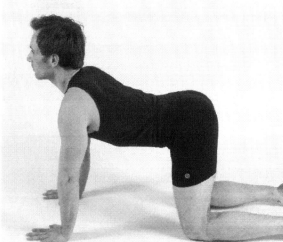

Cobra Variation

Lie face down, and instead of trying to straighten your arms fully by locking your elbows, balance on your forearms. This way you prevent hyperextension in case you have a spinal anomaly that would worsen if you extend too far back.

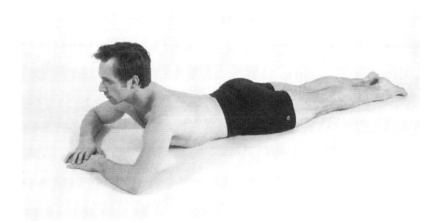

Spinal Twist: Ardha Matsyendrasana

This stretch is similar to the spinal erector stretch in my essential 5 stretches as well as to my spinal twist movement. The only difference is that you perform this one while seated. I generally have no issues with this yoga pose, except that it may result in too much knee tension.

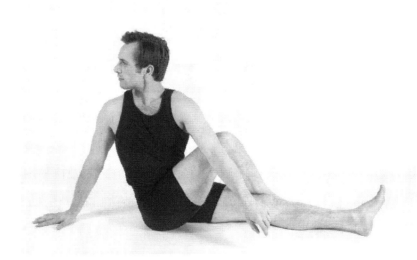

Warrior I

The standing Warrior I pose strengthens and stretches the hips and front of the thighs to provide better support for the back. Begin by putting one foot behind the other about 3 feet apart, with the back foot turned out and the arch aligned with the heel of the front foot. Face your torso and hips forward, bring your arms straight overhead into the air, and bend your front leg without bringing your knee past your ankle. After doing this on one side for three breaths, switch and do it on the other side.

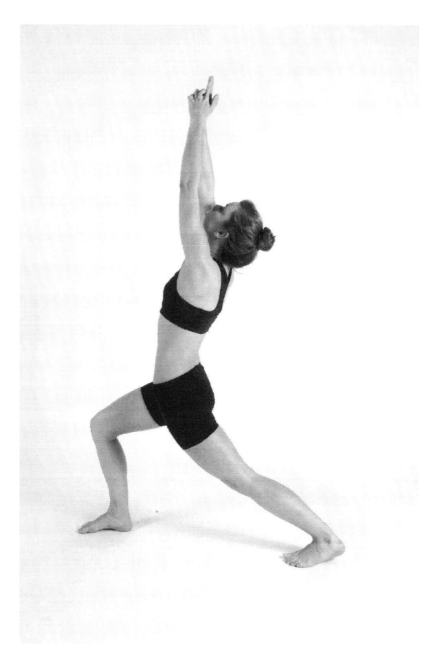

Downward Dog

This pose targets the lower back, neck, hips, and legs, delivering all-around spinal support. Start on all fours, in the same manner as the cat/cow pose. Lift one leg at a time and stretch it behind you as comfortably as you can while also lifting your upper body. Try to keep a straight spine and do not round the lower back. Use your hips as a hinge and think of folding your spine at the hips. The key here is to stay in that position within your limits; make sure that you do not overexert strain to the lower back. Focus on keeping your shoulder blades pressed against your torso, which will ensure a good base of upper body support. While maintaining this common yoga pose, you will also feel a tremendous pull to the back part of your calves while trying to keep your heels pressed to the floor.

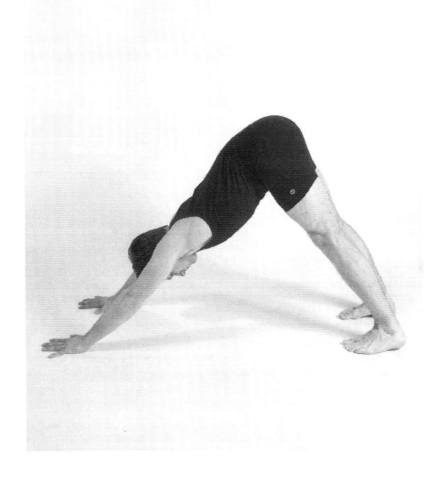

Yoga Poses That Destroy Your Spine

If you have lower back pain, there are some yoga poses you should either not do at all or modify with props. They include the following.

Bow: Dhanurasana

In my opinion, this is probably the worst yoga pose that is commonly performed. I'm not really sure why anyone would attempt it; I imagine the ones who do have always been able to get into a posture like this since childhood. Again, this is generally the type of client yoga attracts. And as crazy as it sounds, this person probably needs yoga to stay limber because of all the destructive spinal changes that have likely occurred from this type of posture.

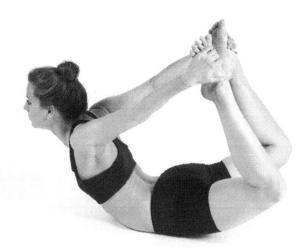

A Cautionary Yoga Tale

Early in my career, a famous yoga instructor who started the yoga trend in New York City health clubs came to me one day complaining of low back pain. We took x-rays of the spine, and to the surprise of this fit 40-year-old female, she had advanced spinal degenerative disc disease and arthritis throughout the lumbar spine. The explanation: she was performing yoga eight hours a day, six days a week—that's 48 yoga sessions a week. That's complete overtraining. Even a good thing can be bad for you; forget about good or bad poses, in this case it didn't matter. What mattered is that she overdid it with this type of exercise program and it destroyed her spine.

Backbend Poses

Backbends are dangerous for those with spondylolisthesis, a condition that causes slippage in the vertebrae, potentially compressing nerve roots and your spinal cord. The pose is also dangerous for those with facet compression and degenerative disc disease. Limit the range of motion and use yoga props when available. Always ask an instructor for individual help.

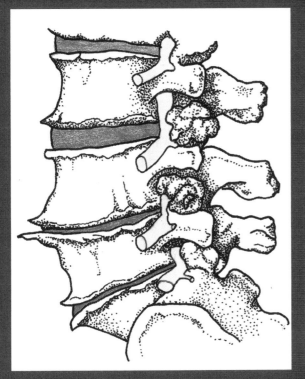 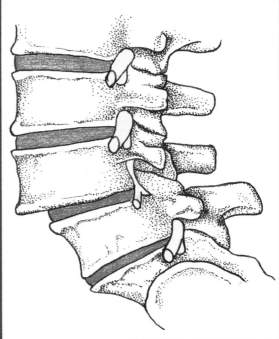

Diagram 6: Arthritic disc compression (left) and spondylolisthesis (right)

Locust: Salabhasana

Like the superman pose, this stretch places undue strain on the spine, compressing and jamming the facet joints together as well as squeezing the sacroliac joints, an action that causes twisting and un-leveling of the pelvis. Remember, this posture could generate over 1,400 lbs of spinal compression. Over time the spine wears out as it can not handle this load on a repeated basis.

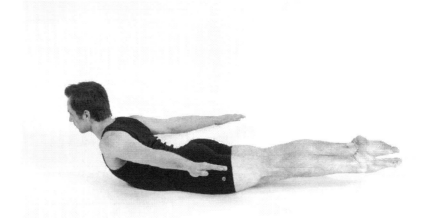

Wheel or Upward Bow: Urdhva Dhanursana

This stretch is horrible, simply horrible. Why bother? This pose offers no benefit to your spine unless your goal is to be in Cirque du Soleil. The fact is, gymnastics wreak havoc on the spine and this is essentially a gymnastic pose, one we probably all tried when we were in preschool. Unfortunately, as we age, this posture becomes so challenging to achieve that injury is more common than benefit.

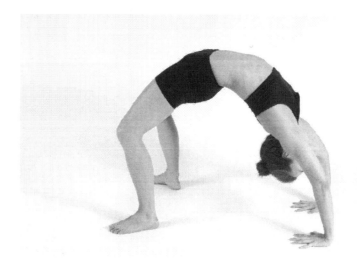

Front Bend Poses

It's all about the time of day with this pose. I would not perform any forward bending in a morning yoga class because the risk of disc protrusion is too high. I also wouldn't perform forward bending following a full day of sitting or after a long bike ride either. The spine is already flexed forward and rounded in posture, which, again, is an environment where the disc is vulnerable to injury.

Recall that during sleep, the spine draws fluid into the discs between your vertebrae, promoting hydration and making you taller when you wake up than when you go to bed. The fatter disks increase the space between vertebrae, lengthening your spine.

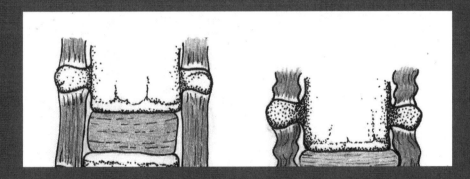

Morning disc swelling (left) and evening disc compression (right)

The larger size means the spinal ligaments attaching one vertebra to another are like an overstretched rubber band, providing less support. This is why, when you bend forward and touch your toes, stoop, slouch in a chair , or pull your knees to your chest, especially in the morning, you run the risk of spine injury do to disk herniations and ligament tears.

To reiterate, the only time I would attempt this posture is following a full day of standing or after a long run.

Standing Forward Bend: Uttanasana
Seated Forward Bend: Paschimottansana

These poses should be avoided if you have a lower back ailment. To modify the standing pose, try standing with your feet slightly apart. You can also try using the assistance of props such as yoga blocks or a chair. To use the yoga blocks, simply place your hands on the blocks instead of the floor. If your lower back is exceptionally tight, use the seat or the back of a chair. Depending on the severity of your condition, you may also want to avoid seated forward bends. Instead, practice downward-facing dog or dolphin pose. (Dolphin is the same as down dog, except you support yourself with your elbows instead of your hands).

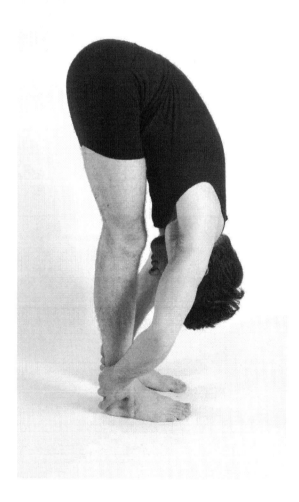

The Plow: Halasana

This one is bad for your neck and low back. I have seen too many injuries throughout my career related to this pose. It is especially destructive if performed after a day of sitting, after a long drive, early in the morning, or after cycling—you get the picture. The potential for low back failure is very high due to the loss of low back curvature; the only time I would attempt this posture is following a full day of standing and if you have no fear of neck injury.

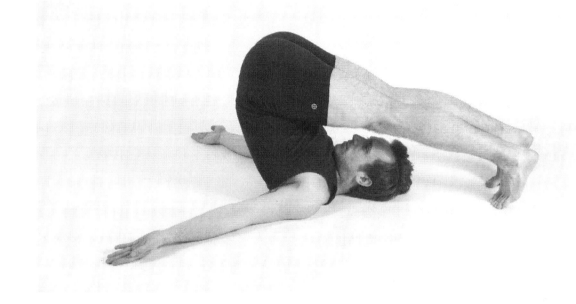

Additional Poses which Harm the Spine

Although outside the realm of detail in this book, I feel compelled to alert you about a few more poses that harm the integrity of our bodies, especially our necks and knee caps:

- Shoulder Stand

- Head Stand

- Reclining Hero Pose

Shoulder stand: Sarvangasana

Though outside the realms of this book, I've had many patients throughout the years who have injured their necks performing this pose. Ideally, this is a chiropractic dream of a pose but a nightmare for the patient. This posture strains the ligaments in the back of the neck and creates an environment vulnerable to disk injury and pinched nerves in the neck. It also sometimes creates a sciatic pain down your arms.

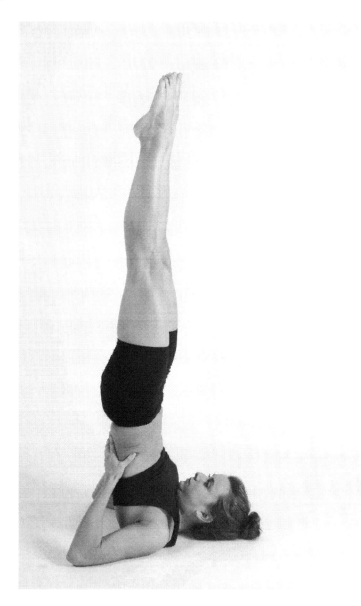

Headstand: Sirsasana

This one should be avoided because it causes too many neck injuries. Why take a chance with the neck? A sprained neck and disc injuries are certainly common results of this pose. I'm not sure what the upside is, as it's a hard pose with high risk of injury. It requires strength and balance; any weakness in the spine could cause you to perform the pose incorrectly, which may lead to a new injury or worsen the existing injury.

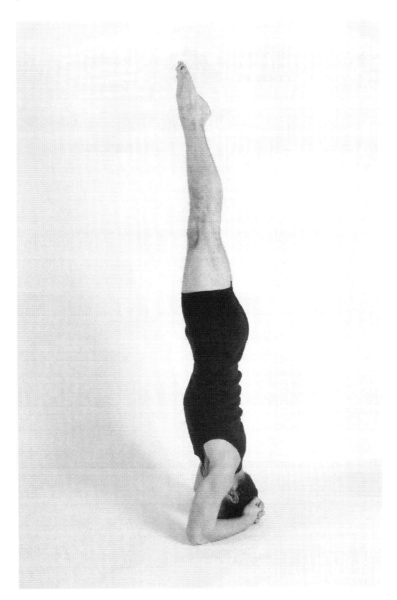

Reclining Hero Pose: Supta Virasana

Avoid this pose entirely. This pose is performed while sitting between your heels and reclining backwards, which puts undo stress and compression on the back. Not to mention that it's terrible for your knee caps.

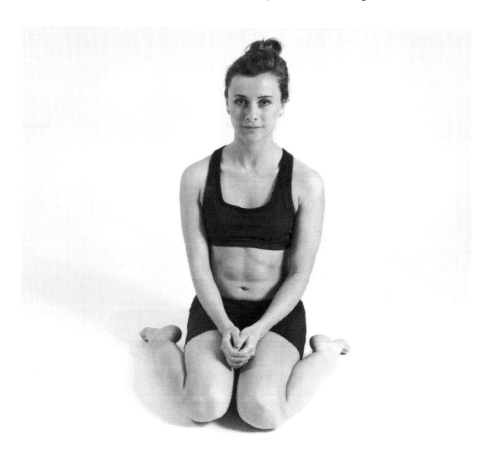

Gyms and Health Clubs

When I first started my practice, I used to train personal trainers at Crunch, Bally's, Equinox, Reebok, as well as smaller boutique clubs. My main lesson was simple, "how not to cause harm to their client." We reviewed biomechanics of the spine and various postures to determine how they related to exercises in a health club setting. Clubs like Equinox have always been ahead of their time and leaders in the industry: it was great to be a part of that era.

That work now continues. I designed this chapter to help clients, personal trainers, and wellness coaches prevent low back injuries in the health club setting. Further, I designed it to allow patients and clients to remain active and safely exercise in a gym while recovering from low back injuries. Its a guideline for them and for you.

I encourage people suffering from low back pain to remain active and weight training is a highly effective activity and necessary as we age. One of the greatest long-term threats to our ability to remain healthy and function independently with advancing age is a steady loss of lean muscle mass (a condition known as sarcopenia). While doctors have long warned about the loss of bone mass (osteoporosis) that accompanies aging, little attention has been paid to the loss of muscle mass commonly seen as we age. Like it or not, we are all aging. We can't stop it, but we can try to ward off some of the effects. Sarcopenia is the age-related loss of muscle mass, strength and functionality. It starts to reveal its ugly head after age 40 and accelerates every decade. It has been shown that 1% muscle mass can be lost per year. Which means, by the time you are 65 years old you will have lost 25% of your lean tissue. Muscles generate the mechanical stress required to keep our bones healthy. When muscle activity is reduced it increases our susceptibility to a loss of bone mass, initiating a vicious cycle of declining health, osteoporosis and our ability to function.

Below are some basic recommendations to keep you engaged with weight training in a health club setting while recouping from lower back pain. Remember, always ask your back doctor if it is okay for you to participate in such activities.

Weight Lifting

There is a common saying which holds true for many people when it comes to losing weight: "If you are shaped like a pear and lose 20 pounds, then you will look like a smaller pear." However, my experience tells me that if you lift weights and lose weight, the weight training will reshape your physique. I love weight training; I perform it four times a week. Further down are some recommendations for those who have lower back pain and want to train with weights. I have kept my advice simple by listing the common exercises that are safe and those that are harmful. It's up to you to decide which ones you'll do.

The reason I do not want you to use weights to train your legs is that lower body weight exercises open up too many ways to injure your back. Instead, back off the weights for the lower body for a few weeks and slowly reintroduce lower body weight training one exercise per workout. This way, if a particular weight training exercise for the lower body irritates your back, you can easily figure out which one it is. Try lunges one day. If you feel fine the next day, then the next time try squats. If you body hurts the next day, you know squats were the cause. Again, if you feel fine the following day, then squats are fine too. Then another time try leg presses; if your back hurts the following day then you know it was the leg-press exercise. Wait a week and try to introduce that movement again until your body is strong enough to handle the load.

Approved Weight Bearing Exercises

Squats

These are great if you maintain a natural arch to the lower back, so make sure you never perform a squat with a flat back. Start with body-weight squats against a wall, then progress to no wall, and then start introducing light dumbbells.

Lunges

Make them stationary and move up and down like a piston. I would avoid forward or walking lunges, as that motion promotes a stooped posture. Recall a stooped posture flattens the normal curvature in the low back, stretching out the ligaments which support the spine. This is a vulnerable posture, especially when under a load of additional weights or a medicine ball. Even body weight loads may create an injury. The downside risks outweigh the upside benefits for sure. All it takes is one wrong move and a low back recovering from past problems will find itself injured again.

Leg press

Perform on the incline and avoid the horizontal leg-press machine, as that position places a stressor on the spine that commonly forces the lower back to flatten and can leave your spine vulnerable to disc injury.

Hanging from abdominal slings

I recommend this tool not to train your abdominals, but to relieve spinal compression that may occur following a weight routine in a gym setting. Use your arms to hang in the slings that are meant for abdominals. Hanging will create a nice spinal decompression that literally opens the spinal joints that are compressed together, like a spring that starts to uncoil. I would do this after every workout.

Weight Bearing Exercises to Avoid

Hamstring curls

If you must do these, perform them while seated. AVOID the prone machine where you are on your stomach because most people who suffer from low back pain have faulty motor patterns that recruit low back muscles before the hamstring muscles while performing this exercise. This means the spine will over arch and compress the facet joints. The facet joints are loaded with pain receptors that when jammed together swell and cause the local muscles to spasm. The above scenario can occur without weights: now load the machine with weights and people generally hyper sway their spine and injure their facet joints. This is one machine I would avoid, especially if you have a spondylolisthesis or sway.

Leg extension

This trains your quadriceps (the front of your thighs). If you have an excessive sway to your lower back or have spondylolisthesis, you should avoid this exercise at all costs. It may recruit too much hip flexion and tip your pelvis forward, exaggerating your spinal curvature.

Abductor machine

This is the outer thigh machine that looks like you are performing scissor-like movements while seated. This machine is problematic in design and set up to cause injury. The person who designed this machine has sent me thousands of patients throughout the years because of low back, hip, and kneecap pain due to IT band friction syndrome. You are essentially seated with legs bent at the knee, which imposes flexion on the hips; then, as you push outward, this outer hip motion isolates primarily the TFL muscle.

This muscle should never be isolated and trained, as it can wreak havoc on the hip joints and low back. It receives strength just from the act of walking, and shortens with the act of sitting, so if you have a desk job it is essentially always tight. If the TFL muscle becomes over-developed, it tightens the IT band, as it is located at the IT band's origin. The IT band runs down your entire outer thigh and has attachments to the hip, pelvis, hamstring, quadriceps, knee cap, and shin. When shortened, it starts to tug and pull on the knee cap, causing tracking problems by pulling it outside of its anatomical groove.

Biomechanically, as the TFL gains strength, it becomes preferentially recruited to performs hip abduction (outer hip motion) and deactivates the glute medius, which is responsible for hip height balance while ambulating (walking or running). This can lead to the development of a hip drop because the weakened glute medius deactivates the quadratus lumborum muscle (which attaches the spine to the pelvis and ribcage and acts as a hip hiker) begins to work overtime in compensation. The quadratus lumborum is a workhorse for spine stabilization and is not meant to move the spine, but as a result of this overcompensation, the QL tugs on your spine until it finally herniates a lumbar disc. Bottom line: avoid this exercise. There are better ways to activate the glute medius for outer hip strength. I recommend a personal trainer (or stick to the basics as outlined in this book).

Dead lifts

Only perform dead lifts under the direct supervision of a personal trainer; my suggestion is to perform them in a bent-knee fashion. Some of the worst herniated discs I have ever seen from gym exercise are those that happened while performing straight-legged dead lifts. Dead lifts are a very complicated movement that requires perfect form. They are designed to train the hamstrings in a closed chain (feet on the ground). This makes it a functional movement for sport. It is a very complicated exercise to perform. I would suggest supervision if you ever attempt this exercise. The biomechanical problem lies with the hinge of the hips with the movement. Either you lock your spine in a sway back posture and jam the facet joints (not great for low back pain suffers), or you lose motor control for an instant and slightly round the low back curve, the results are disastrous. This exercise is not recommended for people with low back pain or weakness due to the high incidence of spinal disk herniations. I see no upside performing this exercise if you have ever had low back pain. It is truly meant for optimizing athletic performance. Unless you are a pro athlete and require powerful legs then the upside is paramount. Otherwise, avoid.

Roman chair

Avoid this one too (see photo on page 17). This is the machine where you lie horizontally elevated, lock your legs under a bar, and flex forward and extend backward. Some people perform this exercise by holding a weighted plate against their chest, trying to gain extra strength to their spinal erectors. I cringe when people do this. It's also horrible to lie sideways on the machine and move up and down in an effort to train their flanks, essentially over training the quadratus lumborum. We already learned what havoc the QL can cause when you try to train it with motion. The QL is a hip hiker and when over trained with this exercise it will distort the pelvis by hiking it upwards, creating a shearing effect on the lumbar disks, which can cause rips and tears.

These are called "annular tears" and when enough tears occur eventually the disk ruptures. Remember, 10% maximum strength is really all that is necessary when training your lower back muscles to avoid back pain. Spinal endurance is the key—not overwhelming girth and strength—when it comes to preventing back pain. There is no reason to perform this exercise. Remember, it creates about 900 pounds of spinal compression (without the chest plate).

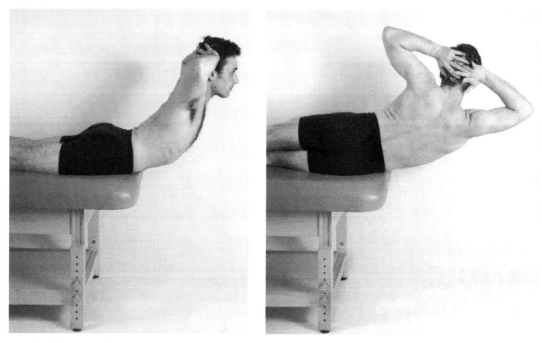

Back extensions (left) place nearly 900 pounds of compression per repetition on the lower back. Roman chair back bends (right) shear the spinal discs.

Abdominal Crunch Machine

I definitely do not recommend this apparatus, the problem is not crunching forward but returning the weight back to the stack. This is called eccentric loading (lengthening of muscles while under a stressful load). The machine places a lot of stress on the low back muscles when reversing the crunch action and injuries are rampant as most people are stronger crunching than extending, the result is muscle strains or tears.

Standing Abdominal Leg Lifts

Again, this machine sets the client up for preferential recruitment of the hip flexors. This means that while "thinking " you are training your abs, you are really overworking your "psoas and quads" the hip flexors. This is disastrous for the spine. Creating a forward tilted pelvis, sway back posture. But worse yet is the "psoas" attach to the front of every vertebra in the lumbar spine except L5 and will exert a compression on the low back joints. Your body learns to use the hip flexors in lieu of the abdominals and abs start to weaken. The result is faulty motor patterns of motion. Avoid this unit of exercise.

Upper body training

In general, upper body weight training in a health club can irritate the lower back. Below are three common exercises that cause or irritate lower back pain:

Overhead presses

When pressing weight overhead, this movement causes the spinal discs to load and compress. If you already have a disc injury, this exercise will certainly worsen it by pressing the disc gel material onto the exiting nerve roots or further into the spinal canal.

Seated rows

Seated rows are problematic, especially when performed on the floor. The client has to reach forward and grab the handle from the cable machine with the knees slightly flexed and the torso bent forward. This posture sets the low back up for failure due to the forward flexed posture and the lever arm which place an enormous amount of pressure on the spinal ligaments. While in this posture the flexion relaxation response occurs—when the electrical activity of the muscles shut down as the ligaments take up the slack. Remember that a spine will buckle with as little as 20 lbs of compression when devoid of muscles and tendon, and in this posture we are relying only on the ligaments to support the spine. When you add the lever arm of weight, the back buckles.

If you want to use this type of movement, hire a trainer and use a different machine, such as one which is seated upright in a chair. The load on the spine when seated upright is much less than when seated rows are performed on the floor.

Abdominal crunches

Finally, avoid any abdominal exercise where you must lock or anchor your ankles in order to perform the exercise. This only encourages the hip flexors to perform the movement instead of your abdominal muscles. The result is preferential recruitment of the hip flexors anytime you try to engage your abs, creating a faulty neuromuscular pattern that becomes ingrained in your nervous system. Remember, the hip flexors attach to the front of your spine and shear the spine into a swayback posture, thus harming the spinal joints and intervertebral discs.

Pilates & Gyrotonics

I like both of these activities for the spine. They are a personalized way to develop core strength in a relatively safe fashion while also providing mobility to the spine. I like one-on-one training when it comes to these types of movements. Ask about certifications to identify a qualified instructor in a health club or boutique setting, then try a few sessions. Avoid a group or class setting until you become familiar with this style of exercise. This way you learn which exercises feel good versus which may provoke low back pain.

Pilates is named after its founder, Joseph Pilates, a German-born sportsman who devised the exercise method 75 years ago, initially to improve strength. It seeks to develop controlled movement from a strong core by using a range of apparatuses to guide and train the body. Originally a mat class of 34 movements, most Pilates classes are held with personalized attention, a trainer, and the use of machines that use springs as resistance. Contemporary methods use props including foam rollers, medicine balls, and resistance bands. The overall idea behind Pilates is energy, flowing movement outward from a strong core.

Many of Pilates' followers are under the impression that the exercise cures low back pain. The truth is that there is little scientific evidence regarding the benefits of Pilates-based exercises for those who have back pain. Participants are taught how to target the transversus abdominus, positioned deep in the abdominal area, by drawing in their navel to their spine and lifting the pelvic floor. According to Dr. Stuart McGill, a professor of spine biomechanics and chair of the kinesiology department at the University of Waterloo in Ontario, it is this concept of "drawing in" that is the problem. He and his colleagues found that solely targeting this muscle in lieu of engaging the entire abdominal corset is teaching people incorrectly and setting them up for spinal problems. Injury often occurs because students are not taught how to do the moves properly. I further find that many people engage the hip flexors and TFL in lieu of abdominal activation, leading again to lower back problems. Even for those who do perform the core contraction correctly, the benefits are good for posture but dubious for relieving low back pain.

That said, I do like Pilates as a way to exercise. Its concepts are old-fashioned, but not truly disastrous to the spine. Don't use it to cure back pain, but if it can get you active and working on an upright posture, then it's worth a try. Professors at the Washington University School of Medicine recently found that, no matter how many times a Pilates movement is repeated, it does not become second nature and therefore will not provide constant back support. Like I suggested earlier, core activation takes practice and it's cognitive, meaning you have to think about it. According to an article in the Journal of Chiropractic Medicine (Miyamoto and Costa 2011), exercise programs for the general conditioning, strength, and endurance of spinal musculature (like the program I described earlier) aid more in the reduction of back pain than any one style of class or training.

Gyrotonic Method

This method employs exercises that use specialized equipment to strengthen muscles while mobilizing and conditioning joints. Key principles employ ballet, swimming, gymnastics, and yoga. Fluid in motion, it was originally developed by Julia Horvath as a way to heal injuries that she sustained from a professional dance career. The equipment uses pulley towers and creates fluidity and smoothness through gentle, seamless movement that can be used as an aid in healing injuries.

I'm a fan, for I find the gyrotonic method to be compatible with people who have back pain. The problem is that it requires personal training, and it is challenging to find qualified instructors nearby. Again, check certifications and avoid a class setting until you learn the methods and movements. It won't be long until someone opens a shop and calls it "power-gyro," so be certain to check credentials before hiring a trainer. It doesn't cure back pain, but it doesn't cause it either.

Massage

Massage is the manipulation of superficial and deeper layers of muscle and connective tissue to enhance function, aid in the healing process, and promote relaxation and wellbeing. In my practice, I treat patients by the manipulation of soft tissue using Active Release (www.activerelease.com), a specific method utilizing hundreds of patented hands-on protocols to release adhesions and scarred tissue that prohibits functional motion. It's the specificity of finding the precise anatomy that isolates movements that makes this technique invaluable to those with soft tissue injuries.

I also use a technique known as Graston (www.grastontechnique.com), which uses handheld instruments to penetrate into deep fasciae. Patented in design, these stainless steel instruments help the doctor alleviate deeper scarred tissue adhesions from old injuries or past surgical procedures, such as deep within a joint space like those that develop from hip replacement surgery. We manipulate joints, muscles, ligaments, fasciae, tendons, and nerves using manual contact for tension and the motion of the affected tissues to produce changes in texture, tension, movement, and function. It is the type of contact and motion of the body that distinguishes our techniques. However, I recommend massage to patients as another component of healing. Again, it's not a cure-all, but it helps with low back pain, especially if they target the right areas. I suggest you tell the therapist to place a bolster under your abdomen, not under your knees (as is commonly practiced). This will help prevent sway

Dr. Duke Rx for Massage
(approximately 60 minute session)

This is a list of specific anatomical sites which respond favorably to massage to help relieve low back pain.

A licensed massage therapist should be familiar with my selection. If not, find yourself another masseuse!

Please target the following tissues:

- piriformis
- tensor fascae latae
- IT band
- glute medius and minimus
- dorsal sacral fascae
- quadratus lumborum at the iliac crest and transverse process of lumbar spine
- rectus femoris at iliac crest
- adductors
- psoas insertion
- psoas midbelly

Ahhh—relief!

back while lying face down. Also suggest the therapist not press too deeply, thereby avoiding compression and tissue damage. Often clients use massage as a way to alleviate back pain, not realizing their back muscles are swollen. They think deep pressure will help the spasm, but end up in more pain after the massage than before it. For your convenience, I have provided a list of muscles I recommend massage therapists target as a way to help patients with lower back pain.

Cycling, Triathlons, Spin Classes, and Lower Back Pain

A lot of us are moving—and that's good news. The best estimates show that there are about one billion people in the world who own a bicycle. The number of Americans who ride bicycles is greater than all those who ski, golf, and play tennis combined. Approximately fifty seven million people over the age of sixteen ride a bike at least one time during the summer in the United States. I join the more than 200,000 people who bike every day in Manhattan.

For years, the National Sporting Goods Association (NSGA) has been conducting surveys of the U.S. population to see how many people are participating in what sports and how often. From aerobics, badminton, skateboarding, tennis, and golf to ice-skating, lacrosse, hunting, sailing, football, and bowling—the list goes on. The most recent NSGA study—released in 2012—tells us that an estimated two million Americans participated in at least one triathlon in 2012.

In addition, it is estimated that 1.8 million people take a spin class each year. Spinning, an intense workout that can burn a lot of calories, hit the fitness scene in the 1990s. It became popular due to its high activity level and because it is easy to learn. Spinning does not require any dance moves and is non-weight bearing, so it can be a good cross-training activity for runners. Spinning's second generation, which is currently experiencing a renaissance, marries athleticism, music, and inspiring mantras borrowed from the yoga world. The result is a cardio workout tailored to those in their 30s and up who want sweaty intensity without the joint-pounding that accompanies running.

While large corporate gyms have responded by putting out spin studios with new high-performance stationary bikes, the race for indoor-cycling dominance is taking place within high-end boutique studios. Soul Cycle and Flywheel are two such studios that are all the rage in New York City. Now, a new fad allows you to spin and lift weights for the upper body while seated on a bike. Fitness magazine reported that a 135-pound woman can burn as much as 425 calories for 30 minutes of spinning, and with an accelerated rate of exertion, it is possible for a woman of this size to burn upwards of 900 calories for an hour class. So it's no mystery why so many people love to spin. However, with all this great news regarding the benefits of cardio health, calorie burning, weight loss, and low-loading to the joints, there is some bad news in terms of injuries, especially to the lower back.

Let me preface the following facts with the point that I truly love to bike and, through my own experience, I am able to offer advice combined with scientific findings. Here's the scoop:

1. Cycling in general creates a flexed, rounded lower back posture. We already know that this reversed curve to the lower back is detrimental to spine stability. This makes you vulnerable to injury. The first sixty minutes following a spin class seems to be the worst time as your ligaments are generally stretched out and non supportive.

2. Cycling overdevelops the hip flexors and surrounding muscles (quadriceps, TFL, and psoas). The overdevelopment of the hip flexor group creates a swayback posture by tipping the pelvis forward. This jars the facet joints, compresses the lower spine, and irritates sensitive nerve endings.

3. Spin classes have four commonly used positions: seated, standing upright, and stretched forward (like speed cycling). They also use something called jumps, which is when you quickly stand up and then sit down again. This movement is repeated many times over and over. The result of this "jumping" can be an overuse of the flank muscle, the quadratus lumborum. This muscle is a hip-hiker and, when called into action, will shear the lower back and cause damage to the spinal discs. Furthermore, when you do not have enough resistance on the flywheel, you tend to sway side to side, and this movement will create an un-leveling of the pelvis. When the quadratus lumborum is overdeveloped, it will take over the action of the glute medius. This is bad. We need the glute medius to keep our pelvis level side to side.

4. Clipping in is important. If your foot is slightly rotated outward, which happens when not clipped in, you can overdevelop or strain the piriformis muscle. When you cycle, especially during triathlons and spin classes, you need to clip your foot into the pedal to protect against this.

Form and Safety

To ensure safety while spinning, ask the spin instructor for a proper bike set up for you. They will know the details of this set up, such as how elevated to make the saddle, how far the handle bar distance should be from your seat, and so on. If you are a triathlete, get a bike fitting—find a bike professional who can make sure you do not externally rotate your hip and strain the piriformis or round too far forward and strain the lower back.

Okay, having said all that, let me reiterate that I love cycling. It's a great way to exercise, build up cardio health and general strength, and lose weight. Spin classes are fantastic in general, and enthusiastic instructors can help keep you motivated with fun music. In addition, training for triathlons is exhilarating; I did four years of triathlon races, so I know from experience. Nothing gets you into amazing shape like performing a triathlon. So how do we prevent back pain and enjoy bike riding? I suggest a dynamic warm up followed by stretching, strength, and foam rolling.

The Dr. Duke Plan for Preventing Back Pain While Cycling

Remember the app that I co-developed called W.E.RUN? Well, on the app, I also created movements to prepare your body for cycling. There's a whole section dedicated just for people who spin or perform triathlons. Below is a sample list of dynamic warm ups to get you ready to bike as well as some cool-down techniques.

1. Dynamic Warm Up to Prepare for Cycling: Do not stretch before you bike, as stretching will deactivate your muscles and make your joints more vulnerable to injury. Instead, do the following:

   - Hip drops and openers
   - Windshield wipers
   - Dynamic hip flexors
   - Reach-backs
   - Rolling planks Point and reach
   - Cat/cow

- Lunge and reach
- Hacky sack
- Hip gyros

2. After cycling, we need to reverse the flexed lower back posture. So, immediately following cycling, stand up and perform the standing arch reset exercise for 30 seconds.

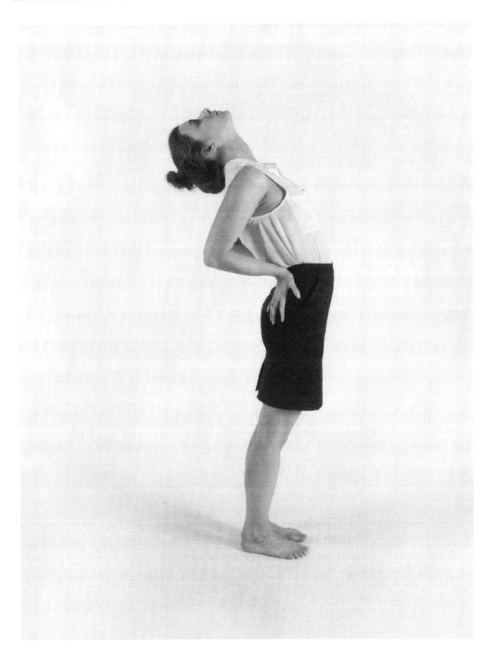

3. Activate your glute medius by performing the single leg bridge for 120 seconds (alternating 30 second holds on each side).

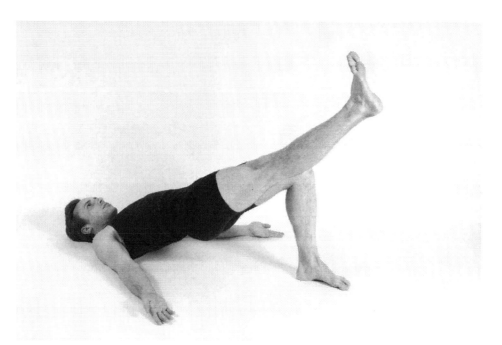

4. Activate your spinal erectors by performing the point and reach for 120 seconds (alternating 30 second holds on each side).

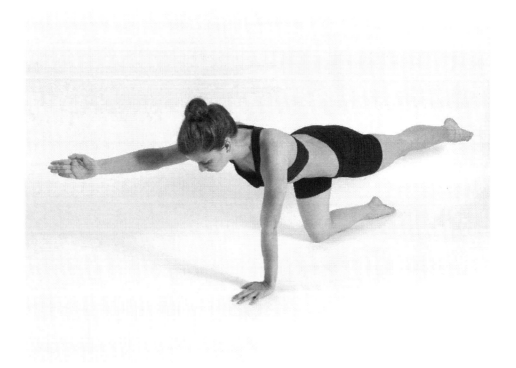

5. Post-cycling stretching: 2 sets each side for 15 seconds each, giving you a total time of one minute per stretch for the following:

Standing quadratus lumborum and TFL stretch

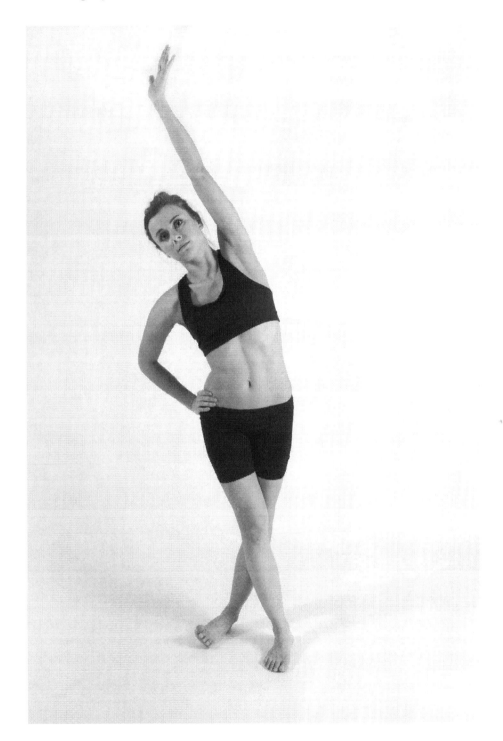

Lunge stretch (hip flexors)

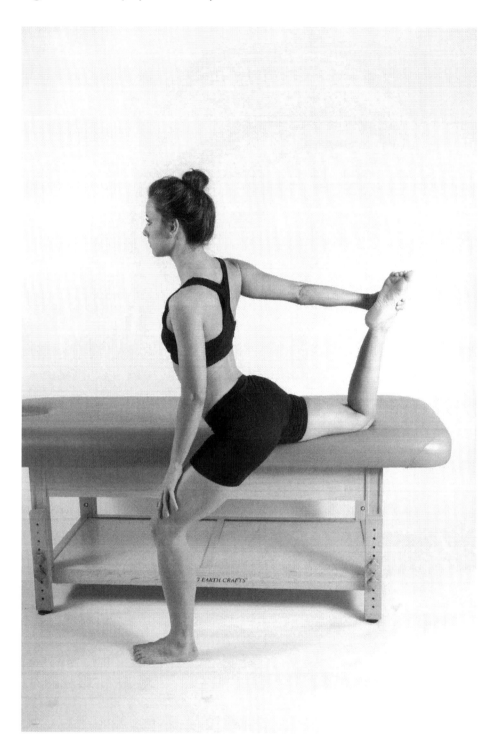

Upper quadriceps stretch

Using a chair, lunge in front of the chair, place the laces of your shoes on the chair, lean back until your heel touches your buttocks, and then perform a pelvic tilt to flatten your lower back. This will isolate the top part of your quadriceps at the front of the ilium and prevent a sway back and tilted pelvis.

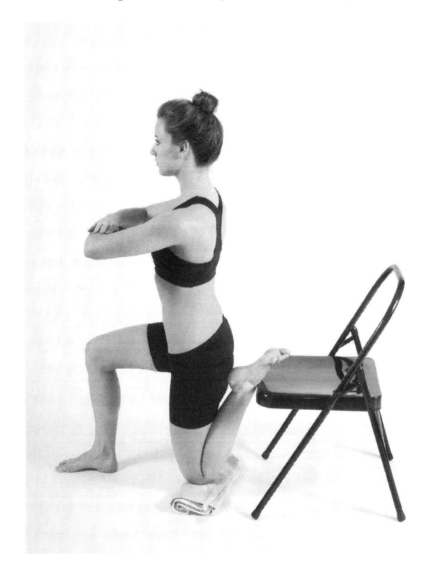

VIDEO 84: UPPER QUADRICEPS STRETCH

The spinal erector stretch

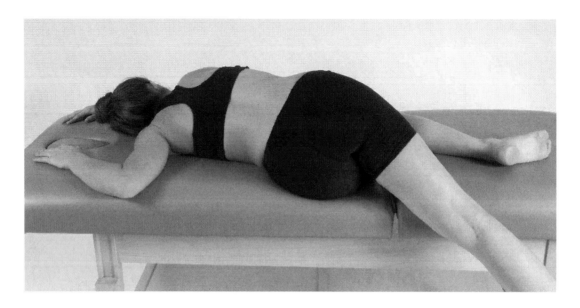

Piriformis stretch

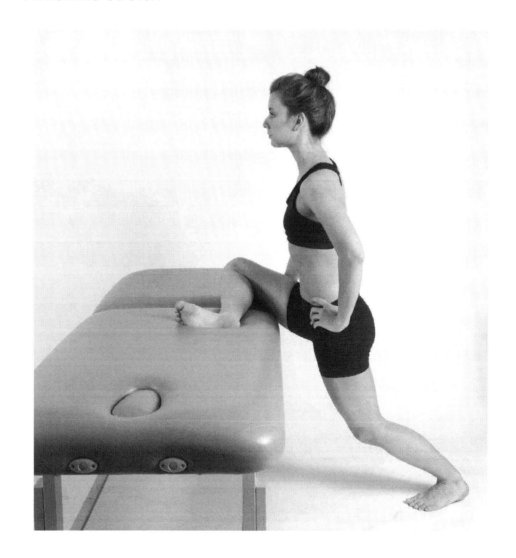

Additional Ways to Stretch the Piriformis Muscle

Piriformis Stretch

The importance of the piriformis muscle (and group of muscles which assist it) can not be understated. When short, tight, or adhesive this muscle group can reap havoc on the spine by distorting the pelvis, creating sacroiliac dysfunction, irritating the sciatic nerve, triggering hip impingement, causing bursitis, etc.

To stretch the piriformis from the floor, lie on your back, bend your knees, and cross your right leg over your left so that your right ankle rests on your left knee in a figure four position. Bring your left leg toward your chest by bending at the hip. Reach through and grab your left thigh to help pull things toward your chest.

Piriformis Chair Stretch

Another easy way to stretch out the piriformis, especially if you have a desk job, is to cross one leg over the other with your ankle resting on the knee of the opposite leg. Gently press down on the inside of the knee and slowly lean forward until you feel a mild stretch in the hips, or gently pull the knee diagonally across and toward your chest.

Foam Roller for Piriformis

Use a foam roller to knead out the piriformis. Cross the ankle of the target hip to lay on the opposite knee. Lean diagonally onto the mid portion of your butt and roll. I included a video to show how to perform this process—a picture is worth a 1,000 words, but a video is worth a 1,000,000! The focus of my videos is to avoid the strain of reading how to move by simply watching to learn.

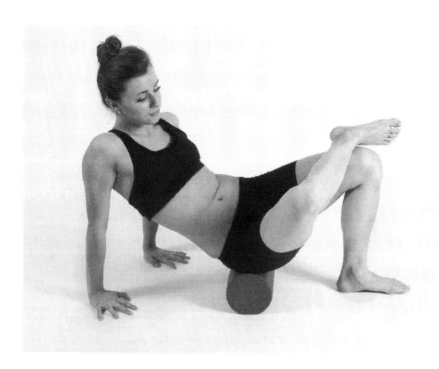

VIDEO 81: FOAM ROLLER FOR PIRIFORMIS

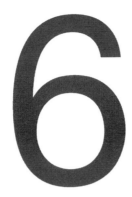

FAMILY MATTERS

"Health is the proper relationship between microcosm,
which is man, and the macrocosm, which is the universe.
Disease is a disruption of this relationship."

—DR. YESHE DONDEN, PHYSICIAN TO THE DALAI LAMA

BACK PAIN CAN AFFECT EVERY MEMBER of your family, young and old, male and female. Aside from the program that has already been described in this book, there is a lot you can do (safe for anyone 13 years of age or older) to help family members prevent and reverse back pain. Here, I will outline a brief guide to back pain for children and older people. I've also included a look at nutrition and back pain, since you are what you eat—and that goes for back health as well.

Children and Low Back Pain

Go to your pediatrician, if your child has spine pain, it's no joke and you need to evaluate the situation. Unfortunately, children are not immune to back pain. In fact, it's clear that the initial onset of back pain is common in youth, affecting one in three children. That's 33%! There is also a marked acceleration in the occurrence of low back pain in children as young as 10. As reported in the American Journal of Public Health, back pain starts early in youth, increases dramatically during the teenage years, and by adolescence, becomes a serious public health problem.

Herein lies the foundation of the cure for chronic back pain: isn't it true that children respond more readily and favorably to back pain treatment than adults? Yes! Shouldn't it be a part of every "well child visit" in a pediatrician's office? I think so. Unfortunately, it rarely, if ever, happens. Does your pediatrician perform spine exams on wellness visits for your kids? Probably not. So, here are basic rules of thumb to follow:

1. If your child has back pain—GO TO YOUR DOCTOR!
2. Check your child's limb length (i.e., see if one leg is shorter than the other). If uneven, ask your pediatrician for a chiropractor.

Most studies suggest that over 80% of children with a history of lower back pain test positive for SI dysfunction (or sacro-iliac malposition), an alignment issue with the pelvis. There is also a good amount of evidence to suggest that a skilled chiropractic physician who performs spinal manipulation is an effective form of treatment for most people, young or old, suffering with acute or chronic lower back pain. Chiropractic manipulation is a treatment approach recommended by interdisciplinary and medical clinical guidelines worldwide.

Children need as much flexibility and strength as adults. Once they hit puberty, they have to be treated as adults in terms of both nutrition and exercise habits in order to help their bodies sustain or handle the load of activity they place on it. The difference between adults and children, however, is that young people think less about injury and seem to bounce back from minor injuries more easily. Think about it—when you were a kid and fell off your bike, you might have cried for a minute, but you got right back on and kept riding. As an adult it's not that simple. A fall from a bike can have all sorts of complications, and you may not have the stamina to get right back on and keep riding. Instead, you may have to run to a doctor because of the possibility of strains and fractures.

As a child gets older and builds strength, their muscles and bones become tighter and more compressed, just like in adults. If they are into sports, they are often doing things to their backs that are very harmful. For instance, I have a 13-year-old son who tried out for JV soccer. In order to do that as an eighth grader, he had to pass the New York City physical fitness test, a very antiquated and harmful test that should be changed but hasn't to date. One of the exercises required are 48 sit-ups to be completed in a minute while the child's legs are held down. This is a terrible exercise for the back; I literally heard my son's hips pull in and out of the sockets with every crunch, and it killed me to watch him train for what I consider to be a useless examination. Since his hip flexors jar the spinal joints and strain the pelvis, it's more of a hip flexor strength test than an abdominal one. It would have been better to have the kids hold a plank position for 60 seconds instead. For all I know, he could have been causing premature damage to his spine. He can do the series of Back in Action routines to counteract this, as long as he doesn't have to do the 48 sit-ups on a regular basis, if ever again. While it's tough to fight city hall on outdated measures such as this physical fitness test, you do have to keep tabs on what kinds of exercises are required of your children and, if necessary, become an active participant in making changes to curriculum if you feel it is dangerous or harmful to your kids' backs or any part of their bodies.

By the way, my son passed the test and yes, I spoke to the coach!

Backpacks and Kids

Pediatricians are seeing a new form of injury in school-age children associated with back strain and overuse caused by heavy backpacks. Often their backpacks equal 20 to 40 percent of a child's own body weight, which is equivalent to an adult who weighs 150 pounds carrying 30 to 60 pounds on their back five days a week. This amount of weight understandably creates strain on a child's spine. Additional strain also comes from children and teenagers who carry backpacks over one shoulder, causing an uneven load on the spine.

A recent MRI Imaging study focused on exactly this problem, shedding light on how disastrous a heavy backpack is for a child's spine. Healthy children with no back pain, aged between 9 and 13, participated in the study. In the study, they were scanned by an MRI machine while standing upright, wearing a loaded backpack weighing 9 lbs., 18 lbs., and 26 lbs. (4, 8, and 12 kgs), approximately 10%, 20%, and 30% of their body weight, respectively. The scans revealed compression of the entire lower spine, T12 through L5/S1, with most of the compression at L4/5 and L5/5 levels. Overall, the L5/S1 disc height was twice as compressed as the discs above it, and the heavier the load, the worse the compression, and the more significant the back pain that resulted. The take-home message here is this: in the adult population, the most frequently herniated discs in the lower back are L4/5 and L5/S1. So, are we setting up our children for future low back problems?

Typically, 90% of U.S. students carry backpacks loaded with 10–22% of their body weight. Add normal variants of spinal anatomy, such as scoliosis and swayback postures, and we begin to exaggerate the abnormal curvatures caused by carrying heavy backpacks. To avoid this, follow my backpack checklist:

- Use a backpack made of lightweight material.
- Find a backpack with straps that are 2 inches or wider, a padded back section, and a waist belt to redistribute the weight from the shoulders to the pelvis.
- Find a backpack with wheels so that it can be pulled rather than carried.
- Look for a bag with individualized compartments instead of just one open sack to distribute weight more evenly.
- Load it with a weight that is 10% or less than that of body weight.
- Pack the heaviest objects first so that they are closest and lowest to the body.

- Fill the compartments of the backpack evenly so that it does not shift while moving.
- Adjust straps so the backpack is snug to body; make the bottom of the backpack 2 inches above the waist and the top just below the base of the skull.
- Do not carry it low beneath the buttocks.
- Do not lean forward when walking; if it is necessary to do this, there is too much weight in the backpack.
- Make frequent trips to a locker each day—don't carry everything in the bag throughout the day.

Pregnancy and Low Back Pain

Back pain problems are so common during pregnancy that they're often considered a normal symptom of pregnancy. In fact, one-third of pregnant women have such bad lower back pain that it limits their ability to work and disrupts their everyday life. If you have a history of lower back pain predating pregnancy, you run a higher risk of back pain occurrence during the actual pregnancy and after childbirth. Due to the strain-related changes that take place during pregnancy, your lower back and abdominal muscles become stretched out and offer little support. You then develop an exaggerated sway in the lower back, which dips your sacrum forward, putting strain on your discs, ligaments, and facet joints. Additionally, you secrete two hormones called relaxin and oxytocin in large quantities during pregnancy. Their job is to loosen the ligaments of your pelvis so that it can expand and allow safe passage for the baby through the birth canal. This functional process creates torque to your spine and strains the sacro-iliac joint, the most common cause of lower back pain during pregnancy. History tells us that if you lead a sedentary lifestyle prior to pregnancy, you have a greater chance of developing lower back pain while pregnant. We know in general that you have about a 80% chance of getting back pain and a 30% chance of it being severe, so why not try and prevent it!

During pregnancy, a good rule to follow is to make sure you don't do anything new that your body is not accustomed to. The point I'm trying to make is simple. If you're a runner and have always enjoyed running, then continue to run while pregnant. But, if you've never run, pregnancy is not the time to take it up.

If you're considering getting pregnant or if you are already pregnant, then please ask your OBGYN before you start my Back in Action program, as you may have a medical condition in which exercise is contraindicated. If you have lower back pain and have tried conventional therapies, including all of the procedures in this book, then seek a referral for a licensed chiropractic physician. Our profession has expertise on providing manipulation to the sacro-iliac joint, the most common area of spinal dysfunction during pregnancy. These treatments are safe and generally offer immediate relief.

Back Care and the Elderly

Let's start with the basics. As we age, our bodies become drier and more brittle, and unfortunately stiffer and weaker too. The fact is that aging causes a degenerative effect on our bodies. We should try to fight these aging effects as best we can, for the sake of our spines as well as our entire heath. Interestingly, however, severe and chronic back pain in the elderly is statistically far less common than it is for adults ages 26–55. The reason for this is that, as I already noted, our discs become drier and more dehydrated as we age, a process that reduces the chance that the interior gel material will herniate and compress painful spinal structures and nerve endings. This is at least some good news for all of us as we age. However, the flip side is that our spines and disc heights deteriorate as we grow older.

Spinal deterioration is one of the most common causes of back pain in older people, as this degeneration becomes more dramatic as we age. Injuries that occurred to our spines early in life usually begin to come back and haunt us later in life. For example, you could have had severe pain associated with a back injury that you never really treated, and once the pain subsided, you were satisfied with the problem. You might have thrown out your back and just waited for the pain to resolve, not realizing that the pain can be gone but the biomechanical problem was still there. Then, throughout our adult life, the degenerative process takes place and, since our discs are dehydrated, we benefit from less pain but probably more stiffness attributed to the aging process. What happened is that a degenerative disc brings the vertebrae bones closer together, resulting in the ligaments no longer being taut but instead slack because of the loss of disc height. The spine does not like instability, so it tries to stabilize using its natural resources and lays down calcium between the bones to try to "bridge" them together. The results are degenerative spondylosis and arthritis. That feeling of stiffness and achiness is no longer related to a back injury but now to a degenerative process that took years and years to occur.

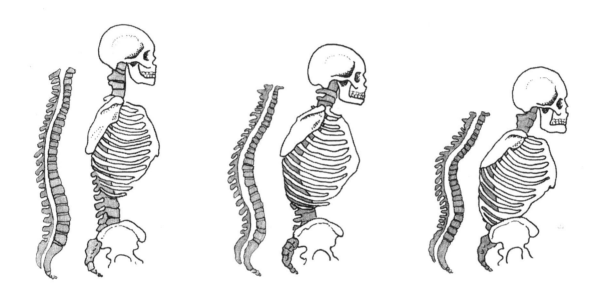

Diagram 7: Degenerative arthritis—side view of three stages

Elderly patients should check with their doctor to make sure that they do not have a serious back condition that requires medical intervention. There are a number of basic concerns to watch out for.

Certain clues raise a red flag that an underlying systemic disease is causing the pain from another condition. A particularly worrisome sign for underlying problems is pain that causes the person to get out of bed and pace at night. Also important is lower back pain that is constant and does not improve over time, which is a clinical sign of spinal cancer: this situation merits additional consideration for problems beyond the mechanical ones.

Signs of serious infection include fever with back pain and problems such as epidural abscesses, septic discitis, osteomyelitis, or bacterial endocarditis.

Malignancy can occur with a number of problems. Prolonged back pain with weight loss or anorexia increases the likelihood of a malignancy, particularly in an older adult with a history of cancer. In fact, lower back pain can be the sign of metastatic disease in an elderly patient with a history of previous malignancy elsewhere. In addition, bowel or bladder dysfunction in the presence of lower back pain raises the probability of spinal cord disease.

Lower back pain may also be related to adverse effects of medications that a person may be taking. Two examples are steroids, which can weaken the bones and may be a cause of vertebral fracture, or anti-coagulants (blood thinners), which can cause a hemorrhage inside the abdominal cavity that may reveal itself only through symptoms of lower back pain. Pretty scary stuff, huh?

Finally, there are psychosocial and emotional factors to consider. Strong evidence suggests that emotional factors are better predictors of lower back pain outcome than a physical examination. Poor lower back pain outcomes can result from depression, job dissatisfaction, or a higher disability rating. It's important to assume a positive attitude towards pain relief. Doom and gloom do not help.

Chronic lower back pain is a common and debilitating problem for older adults. Little exists in the literature about primary MDs acting as primary care physicians for people who have low back pain. Unfortunately, their knowledge of and confidence in managing this problem is not yet favorable. Ask any primary care physician how to manage an acute episode of low back pain and I'm certain the answers will vary from physician to physician. That's part of the reason that I wrote this book in the first place. However, the most frightening part of this equation is the fact that 36 percent of older adults experience an episode of low back pain once per year. Approximately six million older adults suffer from recurrent low back pain and schedule an appointment to see their primary care physician as a result. When back pain becomes chronic, multiple adverse consequences may result, including decreased physical activity and psychological function. In fact, many older adults have non-specific low back pain. For your own personal knowledge, the following conditions can be created, or worsened, by the aging process and may be causative or contributory to the symptomatic expression of pain.

Osteoporosis

Osteoporosis creates weak and porous bones. Therefore, this condition can facilitate easy fracture or even complete spinal instability in severe cases. Vertebral fractures are a common result of low bone density in elderly patients. Compression fractures may or may not be symptomatic; however, when they are symptomatic, the pain is severe. Generally, this occurs from a fall on the buttocks, which causes axial compression, a downward compression that causes the already weakened bone to fracture. As a result, the shape of the vertebrae changes from a box to a wedge, pushing forward and creating a stooped posture. If you have ever seen a person walking down the street with their head flexed towards the ground, you know what I am describing. A wedged vertebral fracture occurred and caused that person to become stooped.

> ### Vertebroplasty
> A procedure known as vertebroplasty can be performed for pain management related to back injury. It's an outpatient surgery in which a pain management doctor injects a cement-like substance into the vertebrae to "pump" it up again. The process is very favorable when tried early on in the development of back pain. Even though it requires diagnostic imaging, orthopedic evaluation, and outpatient surgery, it can be very beneficial for elderly adults. My mother had this treatment after she tripped over a crack in the side walk and fell on her buttocks. The fall wasn't very hard but she couldn't stand up afterwards. It turned out to be a lumbar vertebral compression fracture, but she had the vertebroplasty procedure and the pain immediately subsided.

Osteoarthritis

Osteoarthritis is an ailment that can create pain in many areas of the body, including the spine. It's not a disease per se, but rather a degenerative wear-and-tear process from misuse, non-compliant fitness programs, or excessive exercise. Essentially, it comes about because no one really "flosses" their spine like they should; hence, my Back in Action routine.

Uncomplicated Lower Back Pain

The discomfort in this instance tends to localize in the low back and worsens with stretching, twisting, walking, and bending. The pain causes aching in the buttock or thigh and rarely radiates below the knee. This pain can be relieved by rest and awakened by turning over in bed.

Sciatica

Sciatica occurs when pain shoots down one leg (see page 162 for more details). It is often characterized as sharp tingling, shooting, or electrical pain and may be exacerbated by coughing, sneezing, or laughing—all of which are called Valsalva maneuvers. A common cause of sciatica in the elderly is spinal stenosis, or the narrowing of the spinal canal that typically develops as a person ages and the discs become drier and start to shrink.

Arthritic Debris

Debris-like plaque often develops in the spinal canal and clogs it up, an occurrence that becomes a main source of back problems for the elderly. This is called central spinal canal stenosis. In addition, bone spur formation in the vertebrae may lead to neurological impairment or mechanical pain. Sometimes

If you have leg pain that worsens with standing and walking, but is relieved by sitting or bending forward, you might have some type of spinal canal stenosis. See your doctor and get a MRI to evaluate the severity.

the pain may not be in the lower back but rather down the backs of both thighs. The patient usually develops a forward, slightly stooped posture as this type of posture "opens" the spinal canal thus creating more room for the debris so that it doesn't touch the spinal cord. This person tends to sit often while on a walk to help alleviate the pain.

Degenerative Spondylolisthesis

This degenerative issue can sometimes occur because of severe spinal deterioration. Remember, as the discs dehydrate, they become flatter, the bones move closer together, and the ligaments become lax. Spinal instability is often the result. Spondylolisthesis causes vertebrae to slip forward and backward on each other, causing canal stenosis much like the narrowing of an hourglass. The spinal canal starts off wide, then narrows where the slippage is, then becomes wide again. Mild and moderate cases (grade I and II slippages) are typically not problematic, but severe cases (grade III or IV) may cause serious health concerns and even complete disability in some patients. It often requires spinal fusion surgery.

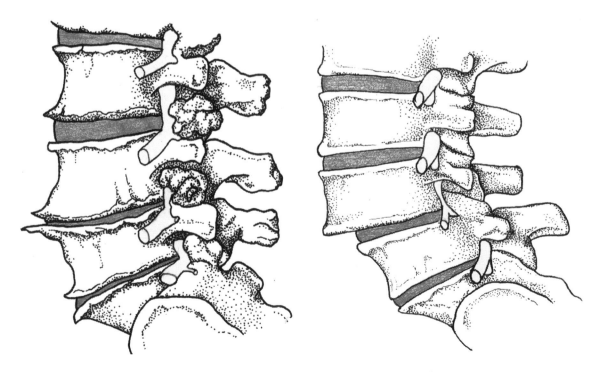

Diagram 8: Arthritic disc compression (left)
Diagram 9: Grade 2 Spondylolisthesis (right)

Scoliosis

An S-shaped curve to the spine is something that people have since childhood. The problem with scoliosis and aging is that as we get older and "shrink," our spines compress, making scoliosis worse. The curve on the convexity of the spine (the rounded part) is fine, but the curve on the concavity of the spine (the inner part) is where problems arise. Bone spurs and spinal curvature, among other possible causes, can create pinched nerves on this inner part of the curve of the spine. Adult scoliosis can result in severe pain from years of wear and tear on the spine. This curvature may compromise the integrity of the central canal or decrease the size of the neuroforaminal spaces where the nerve roots exit the spine, creating pinched nerves.

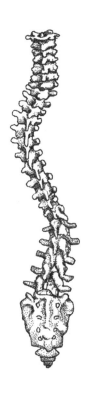

Diagram 10: Adult Scoliosis

A Few Great Movements to Help Scoliosis

A rule of thumb for those with scoliosis: when bending, if it hurts one side but feels good to the other, then just bend to the side that feels good. Avoid doing the exercise on the opposite side. In fact, this is a good rule of thumb with all the movements in this book. Below are movements that are helpful in alleviating the effects of scoliosis.

Full spine stretch

Begin this stretch by lying with the concave side of your curve facing the ceiling, as this is usually your tighter side. Next bend your bottom knee, and keep your top hip stacked on top of the bottom hip. Next, you simply drop your top leg behind you and try to twist your torso so that your chest approaches the floor.

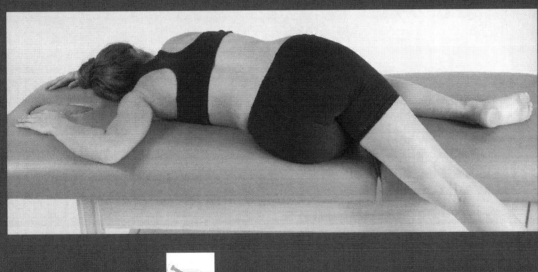

 VIDEO 57: FULL SPINE STRETCH

A Few Great Movements (continued)

Flank stretch

Place your legs wide apart. Bring one arm overhead and reach toward the other side and upward to the ceiling. While concentrating on lifting the rib cage of your tighter side, which is usually the concave side of your curve, take a deep breath in to activate the attachments to your diaphragm, then cross the leg (on the same side as the lifted arm) behind the other leg.

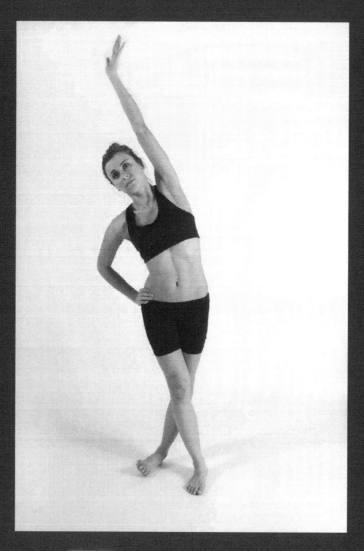

 VIDEO 53: FLANK (SIDE) STRETCH

A Few Great Movements (continued)

Point and reach core exercise

This exercise targets your lower and mid back muscles. I recommend targeting both sides of the spine with this exercise. Remember, you start on your hands and knees and then slowly extend one arm out in front while extending the opposite leg behind you; thus, you are pointing and reaching in opposite directions.

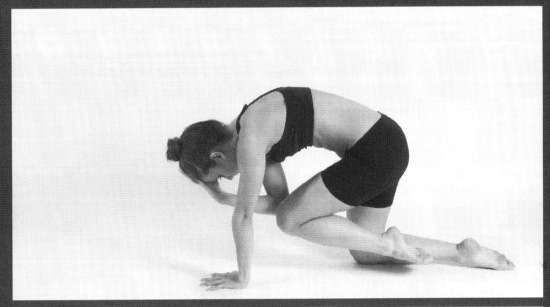

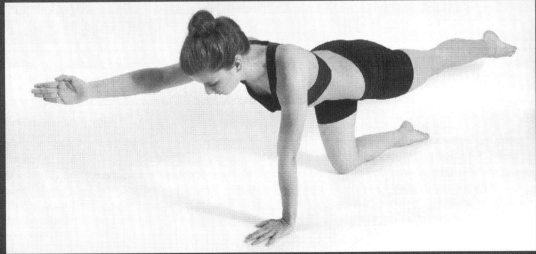

 VIDEO 72: POINT AND REACH

Back Pain from Normal Wear and Tear

Good news for you older adults with lower back pain due to normal wear and tear: there are several *Back in Action* exercises that you can safely practice to reverse your back pain. Follow the routines listed in the book, as most exercises should feel great for you. Experiment and choose the ones that feel the best. If you have spondylolisthesis or spinal stenosis, then avoid extension movements like back arching or lying on your stomach (Cobra), which can aggravate your condition.

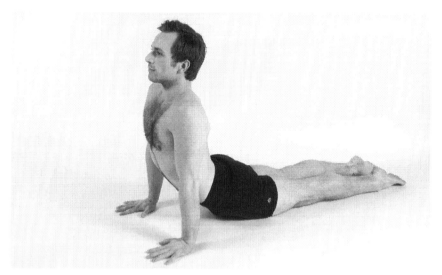

Avoid Cobra if you have spondylolisthesis!

Movements and Exercises to Help Spinal Canal Stenosis and Spondylolisthesis

Except for after a run, the only other time I recommend flexing the spine is if you have one of these two conditions.

The exercises that may benefit central spinal canal stenosis are called flexion exercises. Think of spinal stenosis as you would arteriosclerosis (or atherosclerosis to the arteries of your heart). These are conditions where the arteries clog with debris and occlude the blood supply to your heart and brain, causing heart attacks and strokes. In the case of spinal canal stenosis, the canal also gets clogged, only this time it is not blood occlusion but spinal cord compression. It is not from fatty cholesterol build up, but from arthritic debris. The nerves begin to rub against the arthritic debris causing funny sensations down one or both legs that are relieved with forward bending. The problem with spinal canal stenosis is that there is no pill you can take to help prevent it or clear the canal the way you can with statins for the artery walls. However, there are exercises (or movements) that help open up the spinal canal and create more space for the spinal cord.

Flexion exercises

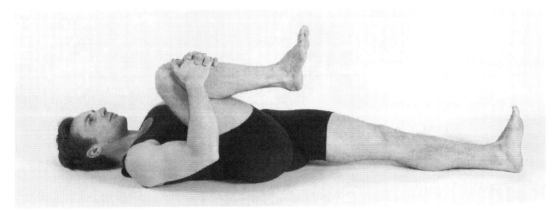

Pull your knee to the chest.

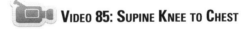 VIDEO 85: SUPINE KNEE TO CHEST

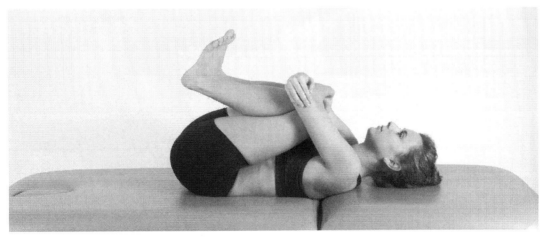

Pull both knees to your chest.

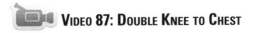 VIDEO 87: DOUBLE KNEE TO CHEST

Prayer pose

Sit on your heels and lean your upper body forward as if you are bowing.

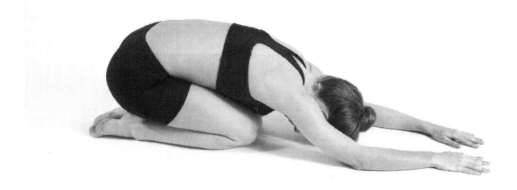

Prayer pose

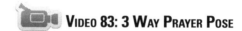

VIDEO 83: 3 WAY PRAYER POSE

While out for a walk, try to sit frequently and, when you do, bend slightly forward to help "open" your spinal canal. This movement will generate more room for the spinal cord, thus preventing compression as a result of the stensois condition.

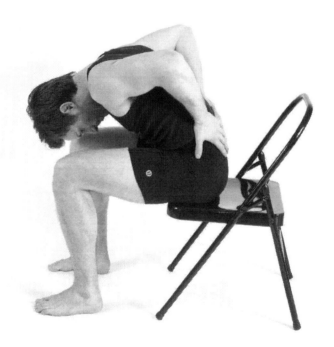

Opening your spinal canal.

Sample Morning Floor Routine
for Spinal Stenosis or Spondylolisthesis

Hip drops

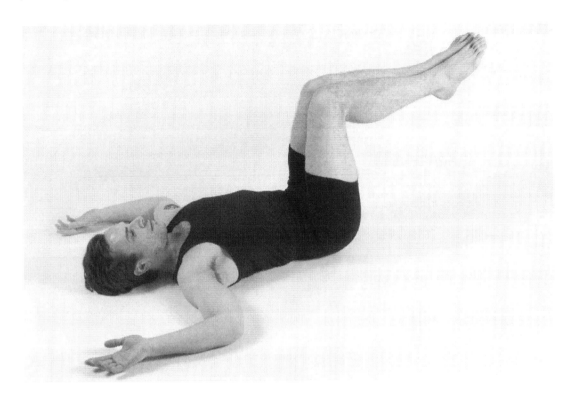

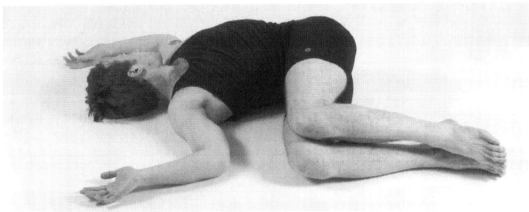

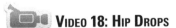 **VIDEO 18: HIP DROPS**

Always perform these exercises on a stable surface like the floor, never on an elevated surface where you can fall.

Lying pelvic thrusts

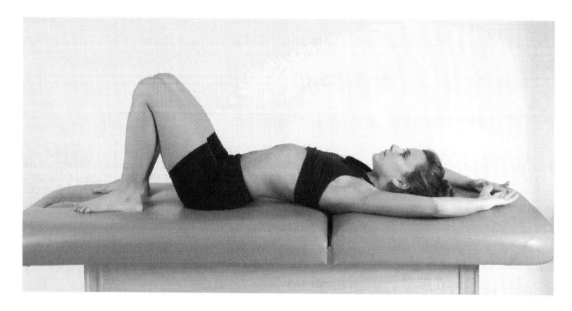

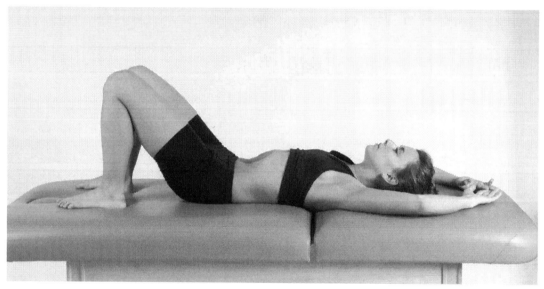

VIDEO 82: LYING PELVIC THRUSTS

Dynamic hamstrings

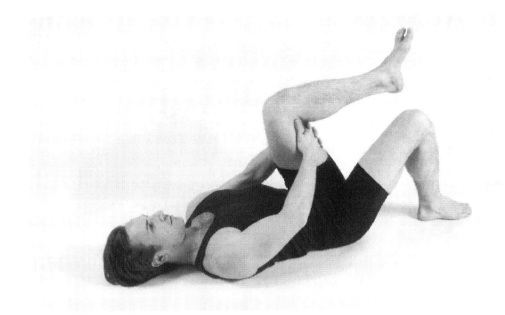

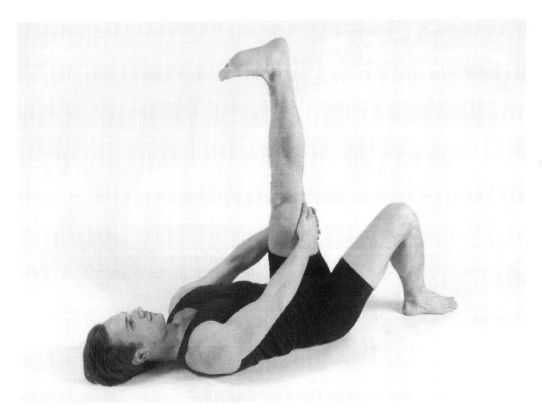

📹 **Video 23: Dynamic Hamstrings**

Hip openers

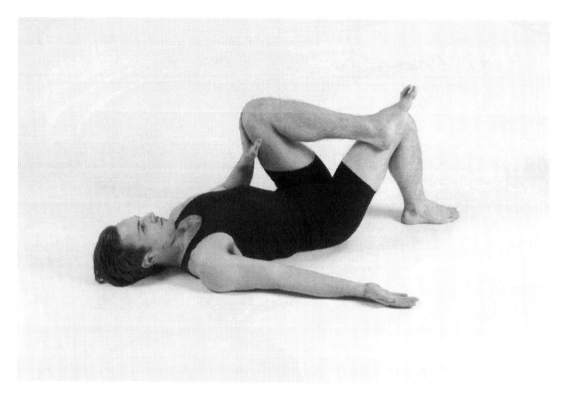

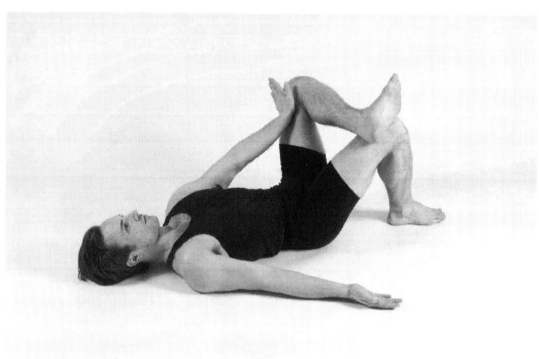

VIDEO 24: HIP OPENERS

Pelvic release

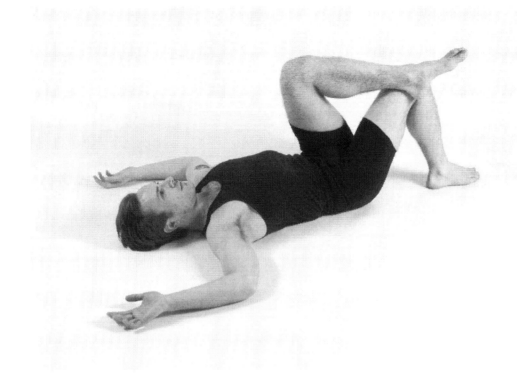

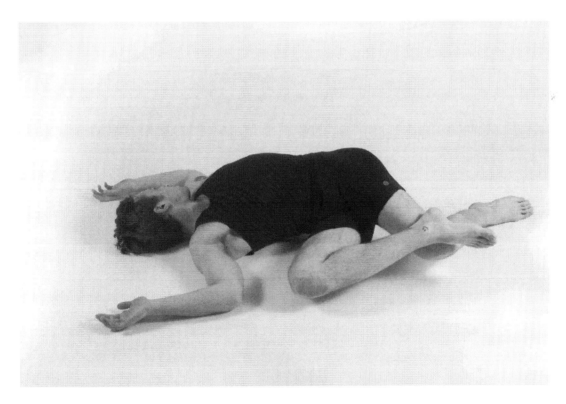

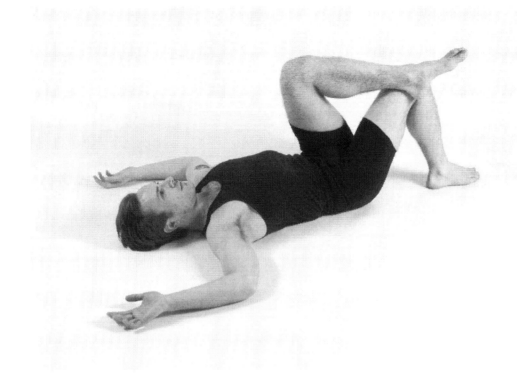 Video 19: Pelvic Release

Dynamic hip flexors

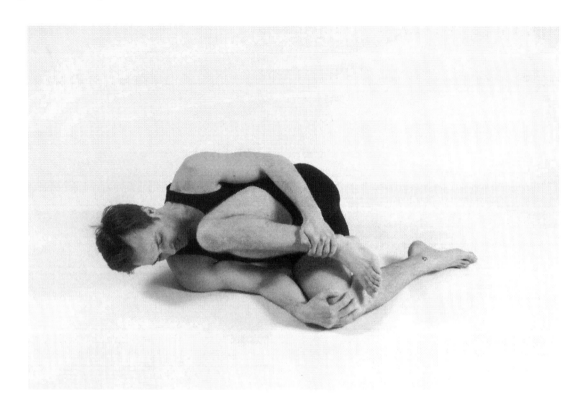

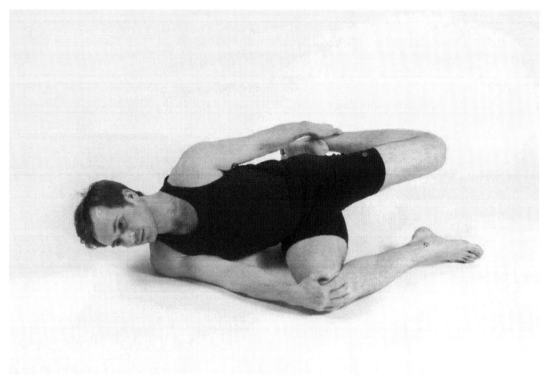

VIDEO 27: DYNAMIC HIP FLEXORS

Open books

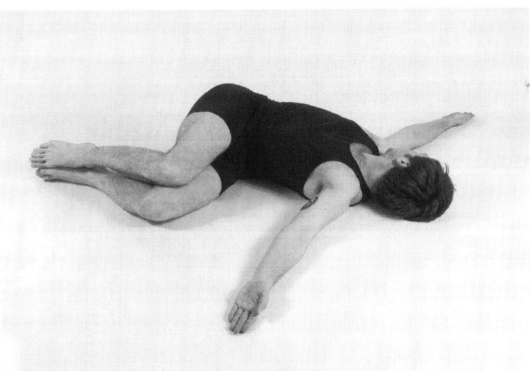

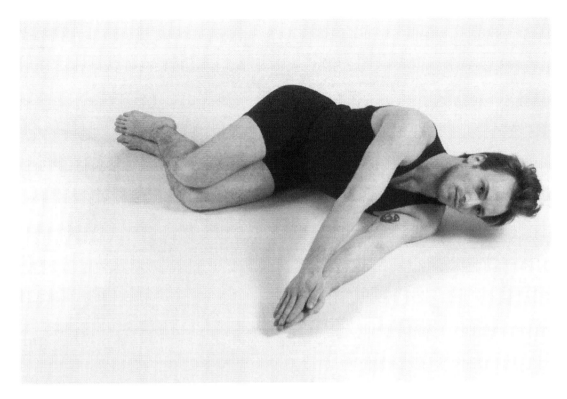 **Video 28: Open Books**

Reach backs

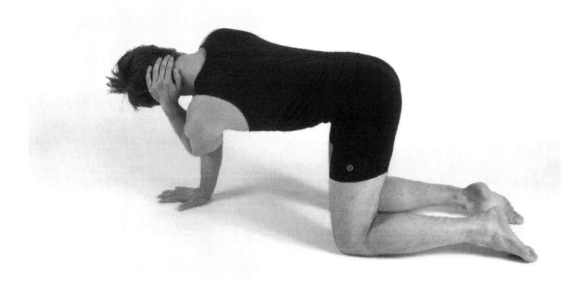

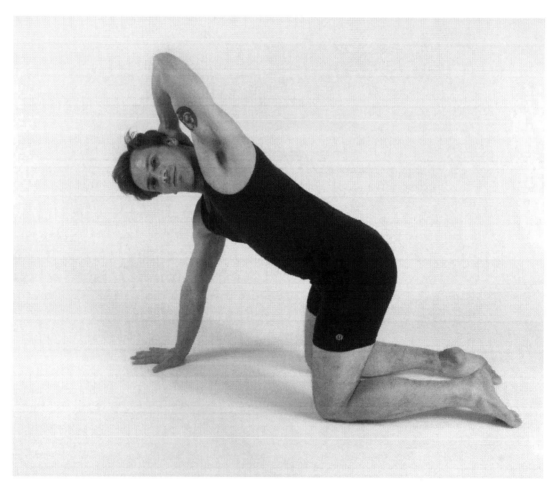

VIDEO 32: REACH BACKS

Prayer or Child's pose

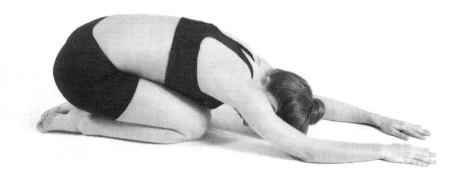

VIDEO **83**: **3 WAY PRAYER POSE**

Cat

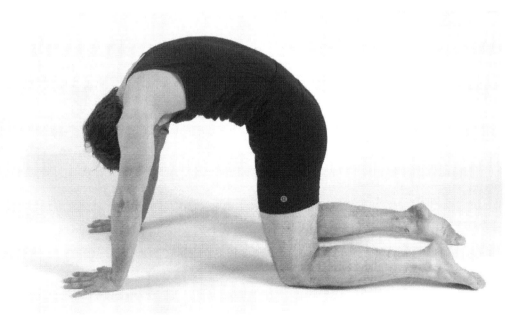

Ab curls to activate your core

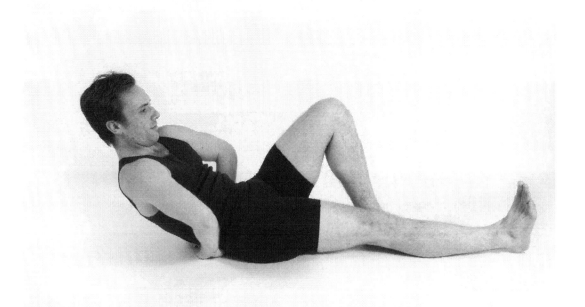

End your routine with some spinal decompression. While on the floor, use an ottoman for 5-10 minutes.

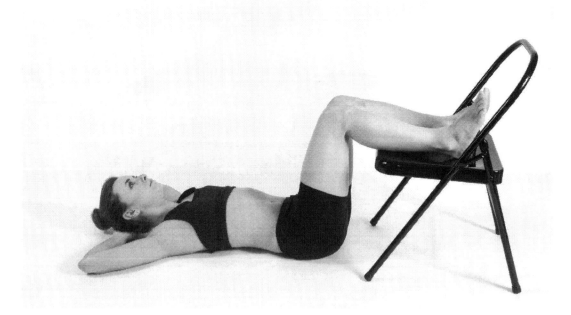

Back and Health Nutrition

Many experts believe that nutrition can have a positive (or negative) impact on your back health, and I count myself among them. A healthy diet that benefits the well-being of your back is one rich in anti-inflammatory foods. This diet is also likely to be suitable for the entire family, and since it's a very beneficial way to eat (low in saturated fats and high in fiber and nutrient density), why not give it a go and see if it helps? I'm not promising your back will immediately feel better by changing your diet—the exercises in this book will give you the fastest boost to your back-health, as well as your general health and well-being. However, over time, an anti-inflammatory diet will support back health. Think whole foods (foods that have been processed or refined as little as possible), lots of fruits and veggies, lean protein, and healthy fats.

Inflammation is destructive to the bones' cartilage lining, the cushion that exists to prevent the bones from grinding against each other. It can affect any joint in the body and is the most common reason for major joint replacement, such as of the hip or knee. It's commonplace for inflammation to affect the spine with pain and disability as well. Since osteoarthritis (which causes inflammation) is thought to be progressive and an inevitable result of aging, research into the benefits of anti-inflammatory foods is paramount for those with osteoarthritis.

Anti-Inflammatory Shopping List

Best Anti-Inflammatory Spices

- ❑ Curry
- ❑ Garlic
- ❑ Ginger (powdered or fresh root)
- ❑ Onions
- ❑ Pepper (black or white)
- ❑ Turmeric

Best Anti-Inflammatory Seafood

- ❑ Anchovy
- ❑ Atlantic herring
- ❑ Atlantic sardines
- ❑ Wild-caught salmon
- ❑ Bluefin tuna
- ❑ Caviar
- ❑ Striped Bass
- ❑ Mackerel
- ❑ Oysters
- ❑ Rainbow trout
- ❑ Roe
- ❑ Shad

Best Anti-Inflammatory Vegetables

- ❑ Asparagus
- ❑ Broccoli
- ❑ Carrots
- ❑ Chives
- ❑ Collard greens
- ❑ Kale
- ❑ Parsley
- ❑ Spinach

Best Anti-Inflammatory Fruits

- ❑ Apples
- ❑ Avocados (all varieties)
- ❑ Blueberries
- ❑ Cantaloupe
- ❑ Cherries
- ❑ Grapefruit
- ❑ Guava

- ❑ Lemon
- ❑ Nectarines
- ❑ Olives
- ❑ Oranges
- ❑ Papayas
- ❑ Peaches
- ❑ Pears
- ❑ Pineapple
- ❑ Plums
- ❑ Pumpkin
- ❑ Raisins
- ❑ Currants

Best Anti-Inflammatory Nuts and Seeds

- ❑ Almonds or almond butter
- ❑ Brazil nuts
- ❑ Cashews or cashew butter
- ❑ Chia seeds
- ❑ Flax seeds
- ❑ Hazelnuts
- ❑ Macadamia nuts
- ❑ Pecans
- ❑ Walnuts

Best Anti-Inflammatory Legumes

- ❑ Adzuki
- ❑ Black beans
- ❑ Black-eyed peas
- ❑ Chickpeas
- ❑ Lentils (brown, green, red, or yellow)
- ❑ Peanuts or peanut butter
- ❑ Red beans

❑ Tofu

❑ White beans

Best Anti-Inflammatory Oils (use sparingly)

❑ Canola oil

❑ Fish oil

❑ Flaxseed oil

❑ Hazelnut oil

❑ Olive oil

❑ Safflower oil

❑ Sunflower oil

Best Anti-Inflammatory Whole Grains

❑ Barley

❑ Brown rice

❑ Basmati Rice

❑ Buckwheat

❑ Quinoa

❑ Oats (steel cut)

❑ Wild rice

❑ Whole grain pasta

Inflammatory Foods to Avoid

When it comes to nutrition I generally leave it to the wellness doctors and integrative nutritionists. However, here are some basic guidelines.

Inflammation in the muscles and joints is often caused by foods, including nightshade vegetables or plants. The most common are tomatoes, white potatoes, eggplant, and peppers. They contain chemicals called saponins which cause inflammation. Many who suffer with arthritis or arthritis-related diseases—such as lupus, rheumatism and other musculoskeletal pain disorders—have found consuming foods from the nightshade family adversely affects their health.

Omega-3 Fish Oils

Alternative research into inflammation has shown that certain dietary supplements can reduce inflammatory factors with few side effects. Omega-3 oils fall into two major categories: plant-derived (from flax or linoleic acid) and marine-derived (from fish). In my opinion, the best natural anti-inflammatory supplement is fish oil. Supplements with Omega-3 fatty acids work in the body to balance inflammation and anti-inflammatory forces. Omega-3 fish oils, especially those high in EPA (eicosapentaenoic acid), can restore the body's balance and mitigate the effects of inflammatory factors. Research shows that DHA (docosahexaenoic acid) and EPA are the most important omega-3 types for health maintenance and that EPA is the most important for controlling inflammation. It was thought that the human body could convert plant-derived flax and ALA (alpha-linoleic acid) into omega-3s; however, recent research dictates that only about 5% of the ALA is actually converted to EPA and none into DHA. The bottom line is that EPA and DHA derived from omega-3 fish oil supplements are the best and most efficient forms in which to consume omega-3s for health and wellness.

Another food to avoid excess consumption of is red meat. Red meat contains a chemical called arachidonic acid, which modulates inflammation. Essentially, it directly causes inflammation in our tissues. A diet low in arachidonic acid and high in omega-3 oils ameliorates clinical signs of inflammation.

Processed foods primarily comprised of simple carbohydrates (like refined grains) are both low in nutrients and full of sugar—detrimental to our health and our waistline. It has been clear for some time that excess sugar consumption creates an improper immune response that leads to swelling and fluid retention in our bodies. Consuming too much sugar can result in binge eating, compulsive eating, and food cravings. It stimulates dopamine and opioid receptors in our brains. These are the same receptors stimulated in people who are addicted to drugs like cocaine and morphine. Stimulating these receptors can become habit forming.

Next are my top 10 foods to avoid because they can cause inflammation.

Sugar

Refined sugar is a favorite food of bacteria and candida (yeast). Sugar is one of the worst foods for those suffering from inflammation because it causes an excess of bad bacteria, which in turn leads to inflammation. Yeast depends on sugar to live and creates toxins that stimulate you to have exaggerated sugar cravings. It's your toxic body full of sugar that makes you reach for that cookie, not your lack of willpower.

Refined grains

Refined grains, such as those found in white bread, donuts, white rice and cereal are not only devoid of necessary fiber, they're packed with synthetic vitamins and artificial ingredients which your body can't process. According to the Journal of Nutrition, consumption of refined grains also causes an inflammatory response because of their high glycemic index (meaning that they cause a rapid rise in blood sugar levels).

Corn

Corn and corn syrup solids can contribute to chronic inflammation because of their high omega-6 fatty acid content. Omega-6 fatty acids are normally part of a healthy diet; however, they need to be balanced with omega-3 fatty acid foods or they can contribute to a host of degenerative health problems.

Partially Hydrogenated Oils and Fats

Partially hydrogenated vegetable oils—such as soybean oil, margarine and shortening—are refined in a way that prevents your body from being able to process them. The hydrogenation of oil heats it at such a high temperature it destroys the molecules on a cellular level. Not only will these oils (and foods made with them) make your inflammation worse due to elevated levels of omega-6 fatty acids, they have no nutritional value and will also make you fat.

Dairy products

Dairy products are problematic because science has turned whole milk into a processed food. To enhance shelf life of dairy products, they are pasteurized—a process which involves heating milk to very high temperatures to kill off bacteria (thus increasing shelf life). However, during this heating, milk's enzymes are also destroyed. Without naturally occurring milk enzymes, dairy is more difficult to digest and many people develop an adverse immune response (lactose intolerance). Because the molecular shape and structure of milk is changed during pasteurization, milk proteins become unrecognizable to our bodies—they are now perceived as foreign and unwelcome. As a result, milk consumption initiates an auto-immune response which triggers many problems in our system, including inflammation.

Cured and commercially raised meats

Beef from cattle fed with grains (like soy and corn) and a diet high in omega-6 fatty acids but low in omega-3s is the most inflammatory animal protein you can eat. Worse yet, to make the cattle grow faster and prevent them from getting sick, they are often injected with hormones and fed antibiotics. This is meat we shouldn't eat.

Cured meats can also contribute to chronic inflammation because they are processed using nitrates. Nitrates send blood sugar through the roof, causing a strong inflammatory response. Therefore, meats such as bacon, pepperoni, salami and bologna should be avoided.

Nightshade Vegetables

Nightshade vegetables—such as tomatoes, potatoes, eggplant and peppers—are usually well-tolerated, but those with chronic inflammation may want to avoid them. These vegetables contain high levels of alkaloids, which can worsen conditions such as arthritis and inflammatory bowel disease.

Dried Fruit

Dried fruit often becomes contaminated by fungus, which can lead to the production of mycotoxins. Fungus, mold and yeast can not only make chronic inflammation worse, they can also contribute to neurological problems.

Soda

Soda can contain two ingredients that make chronic inflammation worse: high fructose corn syrup and aspartame. High fructose corn syrup raises your blood sugar, which may make inflammation worse. Aspartame is a man-made sweetener that has been known to cause inflammation. Additionally, aspartame poisoning has symptoms similar to nearly 100 different physical and mental disorders!"

Fill in the blank

We all have foods that irritate our bodies. My wife, for example, can't eat garlic; when she does, she becomes bloated and gassy and often can't sleep. Many people are sensitive to certain foods but may be unaware of it; they generally brush off disturbances such as tiredness or headaches that can result from particular foods. However, repeated long-term exposure to food that irritates can cause inflammation and lead to chronic diseases. Some common culprits are gluten, milk, eggs, and some nightshade vegetables like eggplant, tomatoes, peppers, and potatoes. The best way to find out if these foods are making you feel bad is to stop using them for a while and see how you feel without them.

The chronic inflammation you're suffering from may be the result of an autoimmune disease. It may also be caused by the food you eat everyday. Become a label-reader and cut processed and refined foods from your diet. Or, seek out an integrative MD healthcare provider or nutritionist.

The Importance of Water

You know that we need water to be healthy, but is water the only beverage that benefits our health? Most whole foods, especially produce, contain water. In fact, you probably get about 20% of the water you need from food. Fruits tend to be the most hydrated, whereas a food such as toast is the least. The other 80% of the water your body requires comes from fluids you ingest, with plain water being the best choice. A good rule of thumb is to consume an amount of water (in ounces) that is 50% of your body weight (in ounces). So, if you weigh 140 lbs., you need to drink about 70 ounces—more than two liters—of water per day. I usually recommend purchasing a liter bottle of water with the goal of finishing it by the end of the day. This way you are at least getting close to the amount you need. Some brands of flavored water have sweeteners, so you need to be sure to read the label for such details. I recommend plain water, with no sweeteners, unless you want the extra calories, artificial flavor, and inflammation with a pre-diabetic boost! I also recommend herbal teas because they have virtually no calories unless you add sweeteners or milk. As for 100% fruit and vegetable juices, they have calories, sure, but they also contain many vitamins and minerals that are beneficial for your health. Watch for some vegetable juices that may contain high amounts of sodium, which has health risks related to blood pressure. Here's an idea: how about juicing your own veggies?

While many people think that coffee and black and green teas have a diuretic effect that offsets the amount of water ingested, recent studies suggest this may not be true. However, these substances do contain the stimulant caffeine, which I do not recommend.

Sugar-sweetened soft drinks like soda are definitely not beneficial healthwise as they have no nutritional value whatsoever. These (even the zero calorie sodas) can lead to excess weight gain. The reasons for this are complicated, but basically the sweetener causes your body to become resistant to insulin (the hormone that regulates carbohydrate and fat metabolism in the body), which is a sign of pre-diabetes.

Drugs and Medications

When in acute pain, there is no problem with taking some style of medication to reduce inflammation. I'm a fan of reducing swelling, bruising, and inflammation. The problem, however, arises with muscle relaxers and addictive narcotics that are masked as pain medications. I do not recommend these because they do nothing to improve your condition, and only help you slur your words, make you drowsy, and create that feeling of wanting more because you are now comfortably numb. I cannot offer you advice when it comes to pharmaceuticals as I do not prescribe them for any of my patients. However, I can provide you with information regarding what the most common remedies are and what they actually do for low back pain—if anything at all—so that you can knowledgeably choose from the myriad of choices your primary healthcare provider gives you based on your medical history. In addition, there are multiple over-the-counter (non-prescription) medications that can be helpful in relieving back pain as well as addressing related symptoms such as inflammation when your back pain is already improving.

Helpful Non-Prescription Drugs

NOTE: THERE ARE RISKS AND SIDE EFFECTS WITH ANY MEDICATION, INCLUDING THOSE FROM DRUG INTERACTIONS. PLEASE CONSULT A MEDICAL PROFESSIONAL PRIOR TO TAKING ANY OVER-THE-COUNTER OR PRESCRIPTION MEDICINE, ESPECIALLY IF YOU ARE ALREADY ON A PHARMACEUTICAL REGIMEN OF ANY KIND.

Acetaminophen

Acetaminophen is probably the single most popular non-prescription medication that people take for pain. It also has the fewest side effects. Tylenol is an example of a well-known brand name medication that has acetaminophen as its active ingredient. Most pharmacies sell generic versions of acetaminophen as well. Unlike aspirin and non-steroidal anti-inflammatory drugs, acetaminophen does not have an anti-inflammatory effect. It's really a pain reliever that works centrally with the brain to switch off the perception of pain. There is no chance of addiction, and patients do not develop tolerance for it. Moreover, it doesn't cause stomach irritation, and very few people are allergic to it.

NSAIDs

Since most episodes of back pain have inflammation as a contributing factor, anti-inflammatory medication, such as a non-steroidal anti-inflammatory drug (NSAID), is often prescribed or recommended as an effective pain medication treatment option. NSAIDs work like aspirin by limiting the formation of inflammation, but have fewer gastrointestinal side effects (such as ulcers or gastritis) than aspirin.

Kidney damage: NSAIDs are cleared from the blood by the kidneys, so it's very important that patients over 65 or people with kidney disease consult their primary physician before taking NSAIDs regularly.

Stomach problems: NSAIDs may also cause ulcers and intestinal bleeding, typically including one or a combination of the following symptoms: abdominal pain, black and tarry stools, weakness, lethargy, and dizziness upon standing.

Three types of NSAIDs are commonly used:

- Ibuprofen (brand names: Advil, Motrin, Nuprin)
- Naproxen (brand name: Aleve, Naprosyn, Relafen, Meloxicam, Anaprox)
- COX-2 inhibitors (brand name: Celebrex)

Ibuprofen (Advil, Motrin, Nuprin)

Ibuprofen was one of the original non-steroidal anti-inflammatory drugs on the market, and is available without a prescription. It is commonly recommended to relieve minor pain, back tenderness, inflammation, and stiffness, as well as some activity-related pain that results from sports, housework, shoveling snow, or other exertions. Since ibuprofen has some aspirin-like effects on the stomach, people with active ulcers or sensitive stomachs should avoid it. In addition, ibuprofen has a mild blood-thinning effect that lasts for several hours, meaning that it can reduce the effectiveness of some blood pressure medications and diuretics.

Naproxen (Anaprox, Aleve, Naprosyn, Relafen, Meloxicam)

Naproxen is available in both non-prescription strength (Aleve) and prescription strength (Naprosyn). It works by reducing inflammatory and pain-causing proteins in the body that are commonly associated with lower back problems. Naproxen thins the blood, so individuals taking blood thinners or anti-coagulants should avoid naproxen, as excessive thinning may lead to internal bleeding. Naproxen also can have adverse gastrointestinal side effects, so people with sensitive stomachs should avoid it. It is best to take with food to prevent an upset stomach. Note: It has had fatal reactions with people also taking MAOI (monoamine oxidase inhibitors) drugs.

COX-2 Inhibitors

This is a newer class of NSAIDs and includes the brand name Celebrex. They work by stopping the chemical reaction that leads to inflammation but, unlike other NSAIDs, they do not harm the protective lining of the stomach. Therefore, COX-2 inhibitors lead to lower and fewer gastrointestinal complications (upset stomach). Also unlike other NSAIDs, they do not impair blood clotting so they are considered safe to take with blood thinners (e.g. Coumadin).

NOTE: NEW INFORMATION SHOWS POTENTIALLY INCREASED RISK OF CARDIOVASCULAR EVENTS (STROKE AND HEART ATTACK) FOR COX-2 INHIBITORS AND, AS A RESULT, THE FDA IS CALLING FOR FURTHER RESEARCH. A BRAND CALLED VIOX WAS PULLED FROM THE MARKET BECAUSE OF THESE FINDINGS.

Other popular brands of prescription NSAIDs:

Toradol, entered intravenously, is usually used after surgery.

Flector is an interesting drug because it can be given as a transcutaneous form, meaning it is administered through an adhesive patch applied to the skin. This is helpful because it means that patients do not need a large dose, which can reduce side effects. It's better to use continuously in order to build up an anti-inflammatory blood level because the efficacy is markedly lower if taken only when experiencing pain. Taking the drug regularly and in the prescribed dose allows it to build up over time and to have an anti-inflammatory effect and a better healing environment.

NSAIDs and Tylenol

Since these two work differently, sometimes doctors recommend they be taken at the same time. Some people report feeling better when taking them simultaneously.

Oral Steroids (brand name Medrol Dose Pack)

Oral steroids are a non-narcotic type of prescription medication that are very anti-inflammatory in their nature and are sometimes a very effective treatment for acute lower back pain. Like a narcotic agent, oral steroids are intended for short periods of time (one to two weeks).

Usually, patients start with a high dose for initial low back pain relief and then taper down to a lower dose. Adverse side effects of oral steroids include weight gain, stomach ulcers, osteoporosis, and a collapse of the hip joints. Due to a possible increase in blood sugar, they are not to be taken by diabetics. Also, they are not to be taken if you have an infection, as they will most likely make your infection worse. Having said all that, I have often referred patients to pain management and orthopedic surgeons to receive this medication when I suspect or know of an acute case of a herniated disc and sciatica. This oral steroid relieves inflammation so well that the pressure is taken off the nerve, allowing me to treat the patient manually and offer self-management advice (like what is prescribed in this book).

Muscle Relaxants

Muscle relaxants are not really a class of drugs, but rather a group of different drugs that have an overall sedative effect on the body. These drugs do not act on the muscles; rather they act centrally (in your brain) and are more of a total body relaxant.

Some doctors make the mistake of prescribing muscle relaxants early on in the course of back pain to relieve the associated muscle spasms, not realizing that the muscles go into spasm to "protect" your spine from further damage. Trying to relax these muscles during this stage generally delays healing, possibly making you more vulnerable to injury. There are several types of muscle relaxants commonly used to treat back pain. Here are a few that are commonly prescribed:

Cyclobenzaprine (Flexeril)

This medication is similar to antidepressant medications. Flexeril can impair mental and physical function and may lead to urinary retention problems in males with prostate problems.

Carisoprodol (Soma)

This drug should be prescribed on a short-term basis only, as it may be habit forming, especially if used in conjunction with alcohol or other drugs that have a sedative effect.

Diazepam (Valium)

Valium is usually limited to two week prescriptions because it is habit forming. It also changes your sleep cycle, making it difficult to fall asleep after stopping the drug. This sleep deprivation can then lead to other drug usage to help you fall asleep, leading you down the road of becoming dependent on yet another medication. Therefore, Valium should not be used long-term. Valium is a depressant and can worsen depression associated with chronic pain. Again, it may lead someone to need another antidepressant drug when all the while it was the Valium causing the depression.

Off-Label Drugs

Is your drug used for an off-label reason? Experts estimate that more than 21% of prescriptions for common drugs are written off-label. According to a study of off-label usage published in the Archives of Internal Medicine, 75% of those off-label prescriptions lacked any scientific evidence to support their usage. The process of labeling a prescription follows. First, the FDA requires that drug manufacturers submit, test, and get approval for a specific use of their product before it can ever be marketed. Pharmaceutical companies must submit extensive research and study data demonstrating safety and effectiveness, a process that takes several years and millions of dollars. When approved by the FDA, the drug receives a "label" for usage, dosage, indications, methods of administration, use in specific populations, along with other details. However, physicians can prescribe these drugs for uses not covered by the approved label, which is called "off-label use." The practice is perfectly legal but lacks any oversight or regulation.

Example: Gabapentin (brand name Neurontin)

This anti-seizure medication has one of the highest proportions of off-label usage for people with back pain. It was originally developed to help patients who suffer from epileptic seizures and pain from herpes. However, Neurontin is now commonly prescribed for people who have been diagnosed with chronic low back pain. Patients should always consider carefully all medications prescribed; it is fair for you to ask your physician whether a drug is prescribed to you for an off-label use. You can thoroughly research this on www.MedlinePlus.gov, the FDA website. It's important to know if there is enough data and anecdotal evidence to support its use in a particular case. Remember, a drug prescribed off-label is a drug that has not been approved by the FDA for a specific health situation.

In 2009, the world's largest drug maker, Pfizer, was penalized more than 2.3 billion dollars as part of a record settlement for violations of federal drug rules, including the marketing of drugs to doctors for "off-label" usage not approved by the FDA. Staff at Pfizer created falsified doctor requests for the anti-psychotic, anti-pain, and anti-epileptic drug Lyrica, a competitor for Neurontin. The drug company essentially gave doctors unsolicited information about drugs to prescribe to patients for off-label use. While it's legal for doctors to prescribe medication for off-label use, it's illegal for drug manufacturers to advertise and market drugs for reasons not approved by the FDA.

Listen, all of this is not to say that the drug won't work, especially Neurontin or Lyrica. These drugs are widely used to treat patients who suffer from nerve-type pain (sciatica or leg pain) and neuropathy (degeneration of the nerves). This drug also may be helpful for those people who continue to have leg pain/nerve pain following spine surgery. It's not well understood why it helps; however, neuroepileptic drugs may be taken safely for prolonged periods of time. They are not addictive, but they do have a list of side effects that is too long to describe fully here. Bottom line is that concerns and warning bells should go off in your head with respect to the safe and long-term impact of drug use that has not been extensively studied and approved to treat a specific disease by the FDA.

Mood regulators

According to the International Association for the Study of Pain (IASP), pain is defined as an unpleasant sensory and emotional experience associated with potential tissue damage. Further, chronic pain is defined as pain that persists beyond an acute episode or beyond an expected time frame for an injury to heal (e.g., three months is considered long enough for back pain to be considered a chronic pain problem). Mood regulators can sometimes be prescribed to help alleviate symptoms of pain, especially in patients where depression results from chronic pain. The goal is to try to stop taking the muscle relaxers and pain medications if you start taking mood regulators. Then work with a toxopharmacologist or a psychiatrist to try and resolve the use of mood regulators so you take them only if necessary.

Cymbalta

Cymbalta was originally created to treat major depressive disorders, generalized anxiety, and to manage diabetic neuropathy. While the mechanism of action is not known, scientists believe its effect on depression and anxiety as well as its effect on pain perception may be due to increasing the activity of serotonin and norepinephrine in the central nervous system. Serotonin and norepinephrine are located in the brain and spinal cord and are believed to mediate your core mood symptoms and help regulate the perception of pain. Cymbalta may worsen glaucoma, cause severe or even fatal liver damage, and result in symptoms of migraines, high fever confusion, and stiff muscles.

On November 4, 2010, the FDA cleared Cymbalta to treat musculoskeletal pain, including discomfort from osteoarthritis and lower back pain. My opinion on this decision is that it's really sad; it's sad that we are resorting to treating pain symptoms with mood regulators instead of trying to offer self-management and healing. Since its initial approval, about 40 million patients in the United States alone have resorted to using Cymbalta to treat their lower back pain.

Narcotics and Pain Relievers (Comfortably Numb)

These are medications prescribed for severe episodes of lower back pain. Narcotic pain medications (also referred to as opiates) are highly addictive. They have a dissociative effect on the body that helps manage pain. Note that I said, "manage pain," not cure or help alleviate it. The body rapidly builds a natural tolerance to narcotic medications so that they lose their effectiveness, making the patient need more and more. In fact, these drugs do not deaden the pain, they simply place the patient "outside themselves" in a dissociated state to become "comfortably numb."

Common brand names:

- Codeine (Tylenol #3)
- Hydrocodone (Vicodin)
- Oxycodone (Percocet, Oxycontin)
- Ultram (Tramadol): While technically a narcotic or opiate, it's different from typical narcotics in that patients do not build up a tolerance with extended usage. Good news for those of you who are interested in staying dissociated from the rest of us.

Who's in Charge?

Who's in charge—the patient, the doctor, or the insurance carrier? There is no question that the excessive cost of American medical care needs to be reined in. There is also no question that insurance companies and managed health care have been ruthless in establishing treatment procedures based on financial targets rather than reasonable patient care. Money that should be going toward patient care is going to a bloated insurance company administration, managed-care CEOs, owners, and Wall Street. In the United States, the ratio of health care administrators to physicians is almost 1:1 (FCER Triano 2008; JMPT: 31:037–643).

Medical research is quoted and selectively used to either exclude or dilute medical conclusions, allowing insurance companies to assert that there is insufficient evidence for certain medical conditions so that they can stop payments and treatments. Basically, it's a significant and inappropriate economic agenda of many health insurance companies. These days, most patients are under-treated as a result of the economically-driven insurance carrier. As health care costs continue to rise, administration and bureaucracy, originally meant to contain costs, have become the problem. There is also increasing distrust among all parties involved (the patient, the doctor, and insurance carrier). The social and economic impacts of under-treatment, if ignored, are significant. Consider this: In 40% of U.S. households, at least one member has chronic pain, and almost half of these people have back pain. (Although this describes the situation in the U.S., there are clearly similarities in many countries.)

Do patients get the care they need? According to the American Pain Society and World Health Organization, NO! People are under-treated and do not receive acceptable standards of care. What happens is that health insurance carriers commonly implement clinical guidelines based on economics. Insurance carriers use rigid guidelines and cookbook rules focusing on a fixed duration of care (i.e., how long it should take to get better) to decide how long they will pay for a patient to be treated. The end result is a totally broken system—administrative costs go up, health care outcomes deteriorate, and everyone gets frustrated. This entire system is inadequate and inappropriate. For reasonable and effective care, rigid guidelines and templates must be reevaluated and replaced. What is not considered is the skill of an individual doctor in providing treatment. Typically, patient actions are totally ignored, as are their beliefs and preferences that influence outcome. Whatever happened to the needs of an individual with personal, biomedical, and psychosocial factors that complicate or delay recovery? Only a doctor—not the insurance carrier—can discover, uncover, and document these findings, interpret what is best for their patient, and individualize a treatment plan. The importance of this is clear and self-evident to anyone who has been a patient.

Think of it this way: appeals court judges are reluctant to overturn a finding by a lower court judge...why? Because the lower court judge saw witnesses, heard lawyers, studied the testimony and faces of all involved, and had the best opportunity to make a decision. There should be a similar respect for and bias towards the doctor's opinion in a patient's health. Most scientific papers do not capture the chronic and episodic nature of lower back problems. If due process is followed, then the doctor's decision-making ability should only be questioned by the patient, not by the patient's health insurance.

Take a vacation!

Ever take a vacation and feel totally pain free? Then, upon your return, all your worries and responsibilities return as you resume life as usual and WHAM, your back pain returns?

The reasons people feel physically better while on vacation are numerous and complicated. Simply put, when we return to a stressful environment (whether our stress is physical or emotional) our bodies respond; for example, many people suffer cold sores, eczema, stomach ulcers, intestinal colitis, hair loss, and acne break outs…you name it, our bodies respond to stress.

Back pain is no different, it's just another area of our body that responds to tension. Our spines respond to physical stress with muscle cramping and spasms. When stressed psychologically our bodies produce a stress hormone called cortisol. When produced in small quantities, cortisol is helpful as it can help us push our bodies to the limit by generating that extra energy needed to accomplish the task. For instance, when pulling an all nighter for work, cortisol levels rise and keep us alert by generating enough energy to accomplish the task at hand. While it can be beneficial for a small amount of time, problems arise when cortisol levels are elevated for extended periods of time. It creates vasoconstriction in our blood vessels—otherwise known as a closing down or shunting of blood from our muscles. Vasoconstriction limits the volume of nourishing blood received by our soft tissue which causes it to become hard tissue. Vasoconstriction causes muscles to become short, tight, adhesive, and then spasm. Only when you finally decompress physically and emotionally (like when on a vacation) will cortisol levels lower enough to adequately rest both your mind and body. This is why people meditate or focus on deep breathing when stressed. These calming activities help keep stress hormones within normal levels. Without calming activities to reduce our stress hormones, they remain elevated and cause our pre-existing physical problems to worsen. Bottom line, vacations or stay-cations are good for us.

Is your pain all in your head?

Psychological factors are complicated in terms of work, family, relationships, and money as they are a plethora of intertwining connections, which is why we have an entire profession dedicated to mental health. You see, pain is very real and the evidence is quite compelling. Doctors and therapists often accuse patients with low back pain who fail to respond to conventional treatment of being mentally weak. The truth is, the medical management team had simply reached the end of their expertise and the failure is theirs—not the patients.

To say that structural problems don't cause back pain is a slap in the face to millions of people worldwide who suffer from it. Back pain hurts and is very real. Torn muscles, scar tissue adhesions, herniated discs, and pinched nerves all have very sensitive pain-receptive nerve endings. When irritated, they cause a cascade of inflammation, which contain chemically-mediated pain receptors.

It's no secret that tension makes back pain worse; however, it doesn't cause it. Tension tightens muscles and narrows blood vessels, this restricts blood flow and results in a lack of oxygenated blood. A buildup of toxic waste embedded in tissue then occurs, further starving the muscles of oxygen. The muscles then develop knots and trigger points that yield pain and discomfort, a condition called tension myositis. However, getting rid of tension doesn't repair the torn tissues that started the "back attack" in the first place. Rather, ridding your back of tension simply takes away the anxiety that suffocates your tissues from oxygen; it's just another tool to alleviate symptoms.

At least now you can be in the driver's seat with the Back in Action method. You have all the tools necessary to successfully heal your back pain, so stop channeling tension internally and start the Back in Action method today. Don't ignore the magnificent advances that medical science has produced. Acknowledge your untapped resource of natural healing and start feeling better today.

7

WHEN TO BRING IN THE BIG GUNS

"Don't ask the doctor, ask the patient."

—YIDDISH PROVERB

IT'S A FUNNY THING being a physician and treating low back pain because it's hard for us to admit that most of the time we don't know why someone is having back pain. It's like you failed and let your patient down when you don't discover the exact cause of their back pain. Patients and doctors alike need answers. This is why in the vast majority of cases doctors who order X-rays, MRIs, or CT scans and see a degenerative disc or herniation say, "Aha! There's your problem. You have disc disease." And then everyone is happy.

Did you know that in numerous studies of the lower back, researchers have found that MRI scans reveal herniated discs and nerve root compression in people who have no back pain at all? It's true; you can have a herniated disc and bone spurs and have no low back pain. Know what else? You can have scoliosis, spondylolisthesis, even arthritis, and have no low back pain. These anatomical variants are found in many people without low back pain.

The problem here is—since most of us will end up with some type of lower back problems at some time—the doctor needs to give you a reason, a diagnosis, or something that explains why it has occurred, or at least enough of a reason so that your insurance company will flip the bill. If the insurance company is not supplied with a diagnosis or a diagnostic imaging that backs up the doctors diagnosis, you guessed it, you—the patient—will have to pay out of pocket for the visit.

Don't feel like you're being held hostage by a herniated disc; it seems like we all get them.

Cat Scans and MRIs

These mechanisms reveal horrible things in "normal" people. Thirty percent of people under the age of 60 have herniated, bulging, protruding, and degenerative discs, but have no low back pain. On the flip side, one can have agonizing low back pain and have an MRI reveal nothing anatomically wrong. So, when someone you know has lower back pain and receives an MRI or CT scan, let them know it may reveal a deformed disc or arthritic change but tell them to be wary when the doctor says, "Aha! There's the trouble." One more thing—there's no such thing as a slipped disc. The discs are sewn to the vertebrae, both above and below, thus making them impossible to slip. If a doctor tells you that you have a "slipped disc," he or she either doesn't know how to explain your injury, doesn't care to explain your injury, or, like most, hasn't a clue what's going on. If this happens, don't walk but run…run far away from that doctor!

Do I Need Spine Surgery?

When treated correctly from initial onset, most episodes of low back pain can resolve symptomatically (i.e., less pain) in about 2–6 weeks.

The National Committee for Quality Assurance in Back Pain Recognition—whoa, what a mouthful—conducted a study in 2006 with 172,000 people who had lower back pain. They were both male and female, ages 18–64, and all of those with "red flags" were excluded (e.g., those with cancer, fractures, nerve damage, etc.), which was about 1% of the 172,000 people in the study. So, 99% of the selected adult population was represented in the study.

Nearly $24 million dollars was spent evaluating and treating these patients. Now, check this out—1,000 participants underwent surgery less than six weeks from their first reported incident of low back pain, despite having no "red flags" (here meaning there was no chance of death or paralysis from their low back pain).

Ok, so less than 1% had surgery. However, here's the kicker—the total health care costs of just these people were $18 million…80% of the total money spent to treat everyone! Isn't it crazy that 1% used 80% of all monies spent?

As a nation, the United States has by far the highest frequency of back surgeries in the world, with 1.2 million spine surgeries per year. That's double the rate of most other countries. In recent years, Americans alone spent $86 billion on doctor visits, testing, imaging, and medications in an attempt to gain relief from back pain. The global spinal surgery market is projected to reach $9.3 billion dollars by 2017, according to a report by Global Industry Analysts, Inc. This is being driven by rising incidences of chronic low back pain, an aging population, and advanced surgical technologies. Yet, at the same time, there is no evidence that Americans have higher rates of back pain than other countries. We already know that 8 out of 10 people at some point in their life experience back pain. In America, lower back pain results in 149,000 lost days of work per year. The annual productivity losses from these lost work days are estimated to be $28 billion per year. So, add up $86 billion in medical expenses and $28 billion on lost productivity, and you get roughly $114 billion spent per year on low back pain. That is totally insane!

In the fall of 2006, the Journal of the American Medical Association published two landmark studies that called into question the wide use of discectomies (spine surgery in which they remove whole or parts of the disc). For the two trials, scientists recruited more than 1,000 men and women with nerve pain caused by herniated discs. In the studies, people chose—or were randomly assigned to receive—either surgery or a combination of non-surgical treatments including physical therapy, chiropractic treatment, and painkillers. After two years, the researchers found that most people felt better regardless of whether or not they'd had a discectomy.

Funny enough, half the people in the non-surgical group switched sides because they felt they didn't have the time to heal. They had physically demanding jobs or small children and couldn't wait to feel better. So, despite the risks of excessive bleeding, nerve damage, and infection, not everyone can wait. People with the most suffering were more likely to opt for surgery, and, after it, they started to feel better in about six weeks. Meanwhile, their peers who sidestepped surgery had receding back pain in about two months.

The point is, everyone ended up pain free. No one should ever feel that surgery is the only option. For those of you who say, "What the heck—sharpen the scalpels, here I come," just wait! There's more to this story.

The exact success rate of spine surgery is difficult to calculate. However, more than 20% of spine surgery cases will have another spinal surgery within five to ten years. Maybe you cured the pain, but apparently the underlying mechanical problem is still there. If you have a microdiscectomy at the L4-5 or L5-S1 level, then 5 years later herniate the disk above or below that level, the protocol is not another discectomy, but rather a spinal fusion. You can not run the risk of having another microdiscectomy because it will generally fail and spinal fusion is the next surgical option that is recommended. It's like changing the tire on your car without aligning the wheels.

A new article from the leaders in spine research states that "doctors and surgeons no longer rely on medical literature for valid and reliable information," but instead rely on industry-sponsored clinical research (Martin, Deyo, and Mizra 2008; Dance 2009). So, if you partly own a company on Wall Street that makes a metal device used for spine surgery, you can conduct your own study and tweak the results, stating that your device helps alleviate a structural spine problem, and then promote sales of the device by writing an article. Sorry to say, but according to U.S. Consumer Reports (2009), spine surgery was recently listed as number one on its list of over-used tests and treatments. The highly respected Journal of Spine Surgery also stated that the current system of approval of drugs and surgical procedures is "broken" (Carragee et al. 2009)!

The bottom line is that prior to surgery, there are plenty of treatment options to try that a quality spinal surgeon will opt for first. Unless it's urgent and requires emergency surgery, it's a quality of life issue. So, the decision is always yours. I'm just here to keep you informed.

Spine Surgery, Scar Tissue & Instability

If you had surgery, you probably needed it. So don't look back. It doesn't matter if you had a microdiscectomy, laminectomy, laminotomy, or a spinal fusion. What's done is done. What matters is what happens now. We need to know how your body responded to the surgery with regards to healing.

In order to perform any spine surgery, one has to cut through and possibly remove muscles, tendons, ligaments, joint capsules, cartilage, etc. The scar may be small but the incision runs deep. Immediately following spine surgery, muscles begin to atrophy, weaken, become non-resilient or elastic, and can rip and tear more easily. They become replaced with a non-supportive, scarred tissue called fibrosis. Next, within five months after surgery, the muscles take on a moth-eaten appearance from this fibrous scar tissue buildup.

After that, there is an impaired neuromuscular reflex, which is when the muscles do not get the electrical impulses needed for stabilization. This, unfortunately, becomes a negative cycle. The more the muscle scars, the less electrical impulses it receives, and the more it weakens. The more it weakens, the less use (and therefore, the fewer electrical impulses) it receives, leading to further weakening. Year after year it becomes a self-perpetuating cycle of low back weakness and injury to surrounding pain-receptive soft tissue structures.

Fundamentally, this loss in integrity to the ligaments, capsules, muscles, and discs that hold the spinal joints together results in a loss of spinal stiffness and stability. You see, spinal instability can both cause and be a result of injury. We need our spine to maintain a certain stiffness to prevent it from buckling.

Remember, a spine without any muscles will buckle at about 20 lbs. of compression. That's all the spine can handle, even with all its ligaments, discs, and cartilage.

This is why I recommend the co-activation of your core muscles (as illustrated within this book) to build endurance and strength not just to the lower back, but also the buttocks, flanks, and abdominals. Strengthening these areas will re-establish spinal integrity and stiffness to prevent further injury.

Spine Stiffness & Preventing Back Pain

This stiffness I am alluding to has nothing to do with the feeling of being stiff and sore. Rather, it has to do with the integrity of your spinal joints in preventing buckling and subsequent back injuries. Think of the following analogy: picture a glass bowl that is very deep and has a marble at the bottom. The steeper the sides, the more stability provided so that the marble cannot get out when tilted. The steep sides are analogous to your muscles and ligaments. If they are surgically removed or are injured (as with an accident, slip, or fall), they become shallower and can no longer provide the stiffness necessary to protect your spine.

Remember, while performing the core exercises recommended, if one side remains weaker than the others, your core will be out of balance. This faulty motor pattern will shear against your spine, eventually causing it to buckle. So, train your core four-dimensionally (front, back, and side-to-side) and follow my endurance guidelines. Get all your muscles to work together with symmetry and you'll create sufficient strength and stiffening to keep your spine safe for all your daily activities. Perform the core program daily until you reach the desired endurance markers and then one to two times weekly to maintain that endurance. Keep in mind the saying "Practice does not make perfect, it makes permanent."

Surgery and Chiropractic Spine Manipulation

Lumbar discectomy is one of the most commonly performed surgical procedures in the United States, now exceeding 250,000 cases per year. I hope your doctor realizes that, unless you have any red flags, like foot drop or cauda equina syndrome, the first line of treatment for sciatica and a herniated disc should consist of non-operative care in the form of lifestyle modification, pain control, careful use of anti-inflammatories, chiropractic care, physical therapy, massage, acupuncture, and local steroid injections. If all these fail after 12–16 weeks, then the more expensive—and invasive—surgery should be considered. Regard surgery as the final option for a solution in what is in many cases a very long journey through failed medical management.

Understand that the well-established failure rate of a microdiscectomy surgery for the relief of sciatica due to a herniated disc is nearly 20%. Similarly, the failure rate of chiropractic spinal manipulation in treating a herniated disc is somewhere between 5 and 40%. Essentially, 60 to 95% of all patients referred to a chiropractic physician for spinal manipulation of a herniated disc receive full relief. However, research data tells us that only 1–2% of patients with sciatica due to a herniated disc receive chiropractic spinal manipulation before surgery.

There is an efficacy of spinal manipulation as opposed to microdiscectomy surgery, especially in patients with sciatica secondary to a lumbar disc herniation. A recent study revealed that 60% of people with sciatica who were not helped by medical management benefited from spinal manipulation to the same degree as if they underwent surgical intervention. People with sciatica and lumbar disc herniations whose conditions failed to respond to the medical management of painkillers, analgesics, lifestyle modification, physical therapy, massage, and acupuncture should consider chiropractic spinal manipulative therapy, and then surgery if necessary.

Your general practitioner or orthopedist should refer you to a chiropractic physician as a first line of offense to help prevent surgery. At least they'll know that if it fails, then surgery is a viable option. But all too many times, a chiropractor is selected as a last option, when a paradigm shift to this strategy of offense may prove extraordinarily beneficial.

Chiropractic treatments fall under the umbrella of non-operative or conservative treatments for sciatica and herniated discs. However, only 1–2% of patients screened prior to spinal surgery receive chiropractic care. Although worldwide guidelines have been established outlining chiropractic care as an appropriate pathway for patients with sciatica and herniated discs, the research tells us that this standardized treatment approach is not usually followed. Furthermore, unless there is a red light for neurological damage, there has been no evidence that a delay in surgery adversely affected the degree of improvement. In other words, try chiropractic manipulation first for three months and, if it doesn't work, then consider surgery.

The options for back treatment are myriad and can be confusing. I hope the information I have provided thus far helps you make some informed decisions about your back care. Mostly though, I can guarantee that with the information here, even if you have had serious back problems for 10 or 50 years, you will finally get some lasting relief. Where you have been failed by doctors, surgeons, and therapists in the past, you can find comfort in your own home with my program.

Collaborative Care

I have met many patients throughout the years who were told that contemporary chiropractic care is not science-based or complementary to medical care. My hope is that by the end of reading this book, you'll be able to reflect upon the sources of your information. Then you'll be able to ask the person who told you the misinformation, "What direct evidence do you have that might contradict the findings of various government-independent investigations, and the experiences of countless MD's who now work in collaborative clinical practices?"

There are approximately 70,000 Doctors of Chiropractic (DCs) Medicine in the U.S. and 8,000 in Canada, with many others also present in over 100 countries and in all world regions. Chiropractic services are now found in the hospital system at Harvard University and at military and veterans administration hospitals throughout the United States. In the past, bias and prejudice existed between the medical and chiropractic professions. This was, and still may be, particularly true where economic interests are at stake, which is very much an issue in chiropractic and medical treatments of patients with the common complaints of back and neck pain and headaches.

Critics of the past suggest that chiropractic treatments are harmful and inappropriate. This is simply wrong. Scientific evidence and current clinical guidelines find spinal manipulation to be safe, appropriate, and a recommended first option for the treatment of patients with neck and back pain. Research shows that 70% of patients who consult chiropractors suffer from back pain, 20% from neck, shoulder and extremity pain, and 10% from headaches (including migraines). There is an emphasis on health promotion and early return to activities with a focus on patient education and empowerment—that is, letting the patient take control of their health and well-being.

Critics have also sometimes alleged that subluxation—the focus of a chiropractic treatment—has no objective existence because you cannot see a subluxation on x-ray. This position is complicated by the fact that modern medicine has a competing definition of subluxation—a dislocated bone. In fact, a chiropractic subluxation is a term that describes abnormal motion involving the restricted movement of a spinal vertebra which affects neurological, vascular, and musculoskeletal function. Since it is a functional problem, it is no more visible on an x-ray than a limp or a headache. The terminology is simply an artificial barrier to understanding chiropractic care for spinal dysfunction.

Chiropractic practice is also regulated. A chiropractic physician has the right and duty to diagnose, as well as perform, order, and read diagnostic imaging (x-rays, CT-scans, MRIs, etc.). Chiropractic education requires an undergraduate college degree followed by four full-time academic years of chiropractic study, then post-graduate clinical training and licensing examinations. Post-doctorate specializations include nutrition, orthopedics, pediatrics, radiology, rehabilitation, and sports injuries. There are more educational programs in other countries (26) than in the U.S. (18). Most chiropractic schools in the U.S. are private while international chiropractic schools tend to exist within the public university system (e.g., Australia, Brazil, Canada, Chile, Denmark, Japan, Korea, Malaysia, Mexico, South Africa, Spain, Switzerland, and the U.K.).

Government and independent medical inquiries have found that chiropractic training is of equivalent standards to medical training in all preclinical subjects. In Denmark and Switzerland, chiropractic and medical students take the same courses for three years before entering separate streams for clinical training.

Evidence-based international clinical guidelines for the management of low back pain recommend spinal manipulation, nonsteroidal anti-inflammatory drugs (NSAIDs), patient education, and early return to activity as appropriate first line management techniques for patients with mechanical low back pain. In short, contemporary chiropractic and medical practices are fully complementary and can be carried out with mutual respect and collaboration.

For acute low back pain, an adequate trial of spinal manipulation is four weeks, two to three times per week. If there is documented improvement, care may continue. Management will typically involve other interventions, such as neuromuscular re-education, therapeutic exercise, physiotherapy modalities, education for self-management, and home care advice. Some conditions require ongoing treatment in the form of medication and physical therapy. This is readily apparent when one thinks of the nature of spinal pain and the impact of continuing with a lifestyle that aggravates the back, or not changing your lifestyle to include safe back habits and exercises to spare your back.

Archives of Internal Medicine published a large study of a California HMO. They found that 700,000 plan members with chiropractic and medical benefits had lower overall health costs per person than 1,000,000 plan members with identical medical benefits but no chiropractic care. Thus, adding chiropractic benefits reduced overall health care costs. People essentially chose chiropractic physicians in lieu of traditional medical care for disorders such as spinal pain, rib disorders, neck pain and headaches, extremity problems, muscle problems, and arthritic issues.

Lastly, to quote the most current authoritative review, "Do Chiropractic Physician Services Improve The Value of Health Benefits Plans?" by M. Choudhry, MD, PhD, Harvard Medical School and A. Milstein, MD, MPH, Mercer Health Benefits (the largest healthcare purchasing coalition in North

America), "Chiropractic care for low back and neck pain is highly cost-effective and represents a good value in comparison to traditional medical care, and is likely to achieve equal or better health outcomes at a cost that compares very favorably to most therapies that are routinely covered in U.S. health benefits plans."

Bottom line, contemporary chiropractic care is safe, cost-effective, and healthy for your back.

Predictive Factors for Spine Surgery

In a major new U.S. study of 1,885 workers temporarily disabled from an occupational low back injury and the factors that predict whether or not an injured worker with low back pain will receive spine surgery, 43% of those who first consulted a surgeon had surgery (Keeney and Fulton-Kehoe 2012). People who first consulted a surgeon for low back pain were nine times more likely to receive spine surgery than patients with injuries similar in severity who first saw their primary care provider. The study goes on to reveal that if the primary care provider was a chiropractor, the odds of surgery were much lower again: "Only 1.5% of those who first saw a Chiropractor had spine surgery within 3 years" (Keeney and Fulton-Kehooe, 2012).

The main purpose of the study was to find early predictors of lumbar spine surgery among workers and "surgeon as a first provider seen for injury" was the main predictor! How crazy is that!

Back pain is the most costly and prevalent occupational health condition among the U.S. working population. Costs relating to occupational back pain increased 65% from 1996 through 2002. (This is only through 2002. I can't wait to see the statistics when they are finally compiled through 2012.) Spine surgeries represent 21% of these costs. There is little evidence spine surgery is associated with improved outcomes yet surgery rates have increased dramatically since the 1990s.

In another recent study from The Spine Journal, a HMO in Michigan called Priority Health decided to address the issue of high rates of spinal surgical by requiring its members to first consult a non-surgical health care provider when first injured (Fox et al. 2013). The results are amazing. Surgical referrals decreased by nearly 50% and resultant surgeries dropped by 25%. That represented $14 million dollars in savings the first year this new requirement was put in place.

But wait, there's more: In a study again published in The Spine Journal and awarded the Outstanding Paper Award by the North American Spine Society, 1,815 patients had spine surgery and 18% had an adverse event occur post surgery, with a combined cost of over $8 million dollars and 4,684 additional hospital bed days (Hellsten and Hanbbidge 2013). In the report the authors note that the U.S. Institute of Medicine's 1999 Watershed Report "To Err is Human" reported that medical errors had an estimated total cost between $17 billion and $29 billion per year in U.S. hospitals nationwide.

The GDP and Low Back Pain

During this past decade there has been a growing amount of research looking at both direct (hospital costs, healthcare costs, medication) and indirect (lost wages, expenses of other family members, expense of adverse events) costs of spinal disorders.

Another recent study from The Spine Journal (the official journal for spine surgery) was made in Australia by a group of health economists to assess the "true cost to the state from lost gross domestic product (GDP) as a result of early retirement because of spinal disorders in people aged 45–64 years" (Schofield and Shrestha 2012; Dagenais and Haldeman 2012). They report that those who retire early because of spinal disorders have 80% lower income, pay 100% less or no tax, and receive 21,000% more government support payments than those employed full time without a disabling spinal health condition. The calculation was huge:

- $4.8 billion lost in annual production
- $622 million paid in welfare payments
- $497 million lost in tax revenue for government and
- $2.9 billion in lost GDP

The commentary explains that these Australian figures translate into a cost of over $85 billion in the U.S., representing a huge economic burden. As an example they use a 45-year-old executive earning $1,000 per day who wakes up one morning with acute lower back pain. They detail the healthcare and other expenditures, which give rise to a total cost of $2,188,595 for the company, 95% of which was due to lost productivity. These economic consequences point to the necessity for a fundamental change in how spinal disorders are managed by spine clinicians.

Emerging Treatments and New Research

Let me leave you with a thought about cures for low back pain. In April 2013, there was a scientific paper published in the European Spine Journal titled "Antibiotic treatment in patients with chronic low back pain." This paper is based on a trial out of University of Denmark, which found that 100 days of treatment with a spinal-disk-penetrating antibiotic was more effective in treating chronic low back pain than a placebo effect where nothing was administered. The lead scientist believes that persistent low back pain in some individuals is caused not by a damaged arthritic spine or disk but a rogue bacteria that has infiltrated it. He found that an anaerobic (no oxygen needed) bacteria was present in 37% of the cases he studied.

Before we begin awarding Nobel prizes and prescribing antibiotics on a large scale let's remember that this was a very small trial study of 162 people who suffer from relentless lower back pain and that two-thirds of the people still had pain after treatment. However, it does demonstrate that physicians and patients are thinking too narrowly when we investigate why someone has low back pain. Nothing is just musculoskeletal or only neurological or psychological or chemical. It makes you realize that everything in our body is integrated and interactive with our environment outside our body. This study demonstrates what I have covered in this book—that factors other than our mechanics, like our immune system, our diet, essentially our lifestyle can contribute to low back pain in ways many people don't expect. In this case, it's a rogue bacterial organism that infiltrates our spinal disks.

Now back to antibiotics and treating low back pain. There are considerable downsides on the potential widespread usage of antibiotics. It's already raised the proliferation of antibiotic-resistant pathogens in both humans and animals to dangerous levels. Antibiotic-resistant bacteria is not the only anticipated side effect: allergic and hypersensitive reactions, GI stomach problems, and dermatologic problems are just a few potential side effects. If antibiotic treatment becomes the norm in treating severe cases, it may not be long before it becomes the norm in less severe cases. As I mentioned in an earlier chapter, it's happened before with surgery, where providers of surgical equipment conduct studies and then tweak the results for their own benefit. Remember, it was a 100-day course of antibiotic treatment; that's no Z-Pack 3-day course. It's not difficult to see some patients demanding the 100-day course and some physicians succumbing to patient preferences. Then it's not so hard to imagine another 100-day course if the first one fails. Just remember this: healthcare in the United States has guidelines but they are voluntary and unfortunately compliance is sporadic. So be careful with new treatments—especially ones filled with excessive antibiotic usage.

8

OUR LAST CONSULTATION

"The next major advance in the health of the American people will be determined by what the individual is willing to do for himself."

—JOHN KNOWLES, FORMER PRESIDENT
OF THE ROCKEFELLER FOUNDATION

AS YOU HAVE SEEN, there is probably no other medical condition that is treated in so many different ways and by such a variety of doctors and therapists as lower back pain. Even doctors of the same profession, schooling, and hospitals have their own twist on how to treat back pain. The fact is that most practitioners have built their careers with specialties focusing on how to manage back pain instead of how to treat or heal it. Pharmaceutical companies and scientists of the 21st century have become intoxicated with coming up with pills in their laboratories to treat the symptoms, but not the causes, of back pain.

Given this situation, patients seek help outside the conventional medical model with alternative therapists with mixed results. They try approaches that promise wondrous miracle cures without any medical foundation. It's such a mess that doctors apparently have forgotten the teachings of distinguished professors, philosophers, and healers who taught them (which is why I mentioned their quotes at the beginning of each chapter). We don't need an alternative medical movement or holistic medicine to recognize the importance of a healthy mind and body.

What we need is a paradigm shift in healthcare—a self-care model of prevention and health promotion as well as a new level of patient accountability. We need to emphasize prevention rather than cure, and integrate medicine and alternative health care disciplines. Unfortunately, we are an aging population with rising chronic conditions. We have unacceptable health care costs and depersonalization in how we are cared for. Worse yet, we employ health insurance carriers who care more about the bottom line than our health.

Patients need to take action and stop relying solely on their doctors; rather, they need to develop an attitude of preventative self-care and take responsibility for their own health. Some of the leading causes of death in 1990, again in 2000, and now in 2013 were tobacco use, poor diet, and physical inactivity. Come on…smoking, donuts, and laziness? Give me a break.

Don't get me wrong—doctors need to take responsibility as well. There is a need for a profound new level of accountability where all healthcare providers focus on quality not quantity, meaning quality of care demonstrated through cost-effectiveness and an adherence to a patient's bill of rights. For instance, a patient's right to make informed decisions with all options available and known.

It's not an easy road to navigate, but if we don't start now, then as we age it will all become more challenging. I mean, do you really want to be reliant on passive care—having someone take care of you and manage your illness—or do you want the ability to heal yourself and prevent illness? I hope that you chose the latter, and that this book has been beneficial to you or a loved one in healing, managing, and preventing low back pain. Keep this book close, read and reread as necessary, and share this advice with everyone you know. As we close our relationship, remember my words of wisdom: "When you hear someone's saga of how they injured their back and that their doctor recommended heat, bed rest, muscle relaxers, painkillers, and exercises that required them to pull their knees to their chest…just give them this book and smile, knowing you just saved them countless doctor visits and probably years of suffering."

It's been a pleasure helping you…good luck in the future.

Best in health,
Dr. Duke

P.S. If you haven't already, I urge you to find a chiropractic physician in your area that is knowledgeable in the areas of soft tissue, diet, therapeutic exercise, and (of course) the spine. Let this physician get to know you, so they can advise you if something related to your musculoskeletal health goes into unchartered territory. My favorite patients are the ones who see me monthly or bi-monthly for spinal "flossing." Just like a dentist who breaks down the unwanted plaque between your teeth to prevent decay, I break down the unwanted debris that causes spinal decay. My "maintenance patients," as I commonly refer to them, are rarely injured, and I am able to provide timely care for things that come up (i.e., physician referrals, review of exercises, diet modifications etc.). Though I am a primary spine care specialist with an emphasis in sport injuries, I co-manage their health with all of their other physicians. So, again, find someone local and start developing your relationship today.

BIBLIOGRAPHY

Texts

Adamany, Karrie and Daniel Loigerot. *The Pilates Edge: Complete Conditioning for Cycling, Golf, Running, Skiing, Swimming, Tennis and Other Sports.* Penguin Group, 2004.

Benardot, Dan, PhD, RD. *Nutrition For Serious Athletes.* Human Kinetics, 2000.

Broad, William J. *The Science of Yoga: The Risks and the Rewards.* Simon and Schuster, 2012.

Chaitow, Leon, ND, DO and Judith Delany, LMT. *Neuromuscular Techniques in Orthopedics.* Lippincott Williams and Wilkins, 2003.

Chaitow, Leon. *Modern Neuromuscular Techniques (Advanced Soft Tissue Techniques).* Churchill Livingstone, 1996.

Chaitow, Leon. *Muscle Energy Techniques.* Churchill Livingstone, 1998.

Duke, Dr. Scott. *Perfect Posture (Crunch Fitness Guide).* Hatherleigh Press, 2000.

D'Ambrosio, Kerry J. and George B. Roth. *Positional Release Therapy: Assessment and Treatment of Musculoskeletal Dysfunction.* Mosby, 1997.

Evjenth, Olaf and Jern Hamberg. *Auto Stretching: The Complete Manual of Specific Stretching.* New Interlitho, Milan 1997.

Gokhale, Esther, L.Ac. *8 Steps to a Pain-Free Back.* Pendo Press, 2008.

Health for Life staff. *Legendary Abs.* Health for Life, 1984.

Heinerman, John and H. Lendon Smith, MD. *Heinerman's Encyclopedia of Fruits, Vegetables and Herbs.* Parker Publishing, 1988.

Jemmett, Rick, BSc, PT. *Spinal Stabilization: The New Science of Back Pain, 2nd Edition.* Novont Health Publishing, 2003.

Johnson, Jim, PT. *The Multifidus Back Pain Solution.* New Harbinger Publishing, 2001.

Liebenson, Craig. *Rehabilitation of The Spine: A Practitioner's Manual.* Williams and Wilkins, 1996.

Lipman, Frank, MD and Stephanie Gunning. *Total Renewal.* Penguin Group, 2003.

Maroon, Joseph C., MD and Jeffrey Bost, PAC. *Fish Oil, The Natural Anti-Inflammatory.* Basic Health Publications, 2006.

McGill, Stuart, PhD. *Low Back Disorders: Evidence-Based Prevention and Rehabilitation.* Human Kinetics, 2002.

McGill, Stuart, PhD. *Ultimate Back Fitness and Performance, 2nd Edition.* Back Fit Pro Inc., 2006.

McKenzie, Robin. *7 Steps to a Pain-Free Life.* Penguin Publishing, 2001.

Morrison, Jefferey A., MD. *Cleanse Your Body; Clean Your Mind.* Penguin Group, 2011.

Rountree, Sage. *The Athlete's Guide to Yoga: An Integrated Approach to Strength, Flexibility and Focus.* Velo Press, 2008.

Sarno, John, MD. *Mind Over Back Pain.* Berkley Books, 1982.

Sinel, Michael S., MD and William W. Deardorff, PhD. *Back Pain for Dummies.* Wiley Publishing Inc., 1999.

Vad, Vijay MD. and Hilary Hinzman. *Back RX.* Penguin Group, 2004.

Waddell, Gordon. *The Back Pain Revolutions, 2nd Edition.* Churchill Livingstone, 2007.

Werbach, Melvyn R., MD. *Nutrition Influences on Illness.* Third Line Press, 1988.

Newspapers Magazines and Reports

"Back Care, What's behind back pain and what you can do to prevent it." Medical Essay, Supplement to Mayo Clinic Health Letter, February 1994.

"Back Pain Treatment Guide." Cleveland Clinic, 2013.

"Back Surgery, Proceed with Caution." *Consumer Report Magazine."* May 2009.

Dailey, Kate. "Stop Doing Sit-Ups: Why Crunches Don't Work." *News Week,* June 03, 2009.

Dance, Amber. "For back pain sufferers, surgery isn't always the answer." *Los Angeles Times,* January 9, 2009.

Garfinkel, Perry. "The Back Story." *The AARP Magazine,* July and August 2009.

Jauhar, Sandeep, MD. "Many Doctors, Many Tests, No Rhyme or Reason." *The New York Times,* March 13, 2008.

Meier, Barry and Duff Wilson. "Spine Experts Repudiate Medtronic Studies." *The New York Times*, June 28, 2011.

Rabin, Roni Caryn. "Screening: Doctors' Group Urges Fewer Scans for Lower Back Pain." *The New York Times*, February 11, 2011.

Reynolds, Gretchen. "PHYS ED- Core Myths." *The New York Times*, June 21, 2009.

Springen, Karen. "To Cut Or Not To Cut, A clinical trial finds that back-pain sufferers with herniated disks improve with or without surgery." *Newsweek*, February 25, 2008.

"When Dealing with Lower Back Pain, Patience May Be The Best Prescription." *WellPoint*, March 2009.

Medical Journals and Reports

Abdi, S., et al. "Spinal Injections Lack Scientific Support" *Pain Physician*, 10 (2007):185–212.

Albert, H.B., J.S. Sorensen, B.S. Christensen and C. Manniche. "Antibiotic treatment in patients with chronic low back pain and vertebral bone edema (Modic type 1 changes): a double-blind randomized clinical controlled trial of efficacy." *Eur Spine J*, 22, no. 4 (Apr 2013): 697–707.

Anderson, P.A., et al. "Randomized controlled trials of the treatment of lumbar disk herniation (1983–2007)." *Journal of the American Academy of Orthopedic Surgery*, 16 (October 16, 2008): 566–573.

Bakker E.W., A.P. Verhagen, E. Van Trijffel, C. Lucas and B.W. Koes. "Spinal mechanical load as a risk factor for low back pain: a systematic review of prospective cohort studies." *Spine*, 34, no. 8 (April 15, 2009): E281–293.

Bolton, J.E. and H.C. Hurst. "Prognostic Factors for Short-Term Improvement in Acute and Persistent Musculoskeletal Pain Consulter in Primary Care." *Chiro & Manual Therapies*, 19, no. 27, 1–27.

Bronfort, G., M. Hass, R. Evans, G. Kawchuk and S. Dagenais. 2008. "Evidence-informed Management of Chronic Low Back Pain with Spinal Manipulation and Mobilization." *The Spine Journal* 8(1): 213–245.

Calmels, P., P. Queneau and C. Haronet. "Clinical Research: Is the Spine Field a Mine Field?" *Spine*, 34, no. 5 (2009): 423–430.

Calmels, P. "Effectiveness of a Lumbar Belt in Subacute Low Back Pain: An open, Multicentric,and Randomized Clinical Stud." *Spine*, 34, no. 3, 215–220.

Carey, T.D., et al. "A Long Way to go: practice Patterns and Evidence in Chronic Low Back Pain Care." *Spine*, 34, no. 7 (2009): 4–5, 718–724.

Carragee, E.J., R.A. Deyo and F.M. Kovacs. "Disc Prolapse: Evidence of Reversal with Repeated Extension." *Spine*, 3, no. 4 (2009): 344–350.

Carragee, E.J., R.A. Deyo, F.M. Kovacs, W.C. Peul, J.D. Lurie, G. Urrúita, T.P. Corbin and M.L. Schoene. 2009. "Clinical Research: Is the Spine Field a Mine Field?" *The Spine Journal* 34(5): 423–430.

Cherkin, et al. "A randomized trial comparing acupuncture, simulated acupuncture and usual care for pain." *Arch Intern Med*, 169, iss. 9 (May 13, 2009): 66–858.

Cifuentes, M., J. Willetts and R. Wasiak. "Health Maintenance Care in Work-Related Low Back Pain and Its Association With Disability Recurrence." 2011.

Colloca, Christopher J., DC, et al. "The Biomechanical and Clinical Significance of The Lumbar Erector Spinae Flexion-Relaxation Phenomenon: A Review of Literature." *Journal of Manipulative and Physiological Therapeutics*, 28, no. 8 (October 2005): 623.

Consumer Reports. May 2009. "Use Caution with Surgery."

Cramer, G.D. and J.K. Ross. "Distribution of Cavitations as Identified with Accelerometry During Lumbar Spinal Manipulation." *J Manipulative Physiol Ther*, 34 (2011):572–583.

Cramer, Gregory, DC, PhD, et al. "Basic Science Research Related to Chiropractic Spinal Adjusting: The State of Art and Recommendations Revisited." *Journal of Manipulative and Physiological Therapeutics*, 29, no. 9 (November/December 2006): 726.

Critchley, D.J., et al. "Effectiveness and Cost-Effectiveness of Three Types of Physiotherapy Used to reduce Chronic Low Back Pain Disability: A Pragmatic Randomized Trial with Economic Evaluation." *The Spine* 32, iss. 14 (June 15, 2007): 1474–1481.

Cruze, R.A. and J. Cambron. "Chiropractic Management of Post-surgical Lumbar Spine Pain: A Retrospective Study of 32 Cases." *J Manipulative Physiol Ther*, 34, no. 6 (July 2011): 408–412.

Dagenais S. and S. Haldeman. "Commentary: Laboring to Understand the Economic Impact of Spinal Disorders." *The Spine Journal*, 12 (2012): 1119–1121.

Demoulin C, et al. "Spinal muscle evaluation in healthy individuals and low-back-pain patients: a literature review." *Joint Bone Spine*, 74, iss. 1 (January 2007): 9–13.

Dougherty P.E. and R.M. Engel. "Comparative Effectiveness of Exercise, Acupuncture and Spinal Manipulation for Low Back Pain." *Spine*, 36 (2011): 8.

Eubanks J.D., et al. "Prevalence of Lumbar Facet Arthrosis and Its Relationship to Age, Sex, and Race; An Anatomic Study of Cadaveric Specimens." *Spine*, 32, iss. 19 (September 1, 2007): 2058–2062.

Ferreira M.L., et al. "Changes in postural activity of the truck muscles following spinal manipulative therapy." *Manual Therapy*, 12, iss. 3 (August 2007): 240–248.

Fox J. and H.J. Andrew. "The Effect of Required Physiatrist Consultation on Surgery Rates for Back Pain." *Spine*, 38, no. 3 (2013): E178–E184.

Fritz, J.M., S.L. Kopperhaven and G.N. Kawchuk. "Preliminary Investigation of Mechanisms Underlying the Effects of Manipulation" *Spine*, 36 (2011): 5, 1772–1781.

Gagnier J.J., et al. "Herbal Medicine for Lower Back Pain: A Cochrane Review." *Spine*, 32, no. 1 (January 1, 2007): 82–92.

George, James W. DC, et al. "The Effects of active Release Technique on Hamstring Flexibility: A Pilot Study." *Journal of Manipulative and Physiological Therapeutics*, 29, no. 3 (March/April 2006): 224.

Globe, G.A. "Chiropractic Management of Low Back Disorders: Report from A Consensus Process." *J Manipulative Physiol Ther*, 31, no. 9 (Nov/Dec 2008): 651–658.

Glu Sabuncuo, et al. "Spontaneous regression of extruded lumbar disc herniation." *Turk Neurosurg*, 18, iss. 4 (April 14, 2009): 6–392.

Gremeaux, V., et al. "Analysis of Low Back Pain in Adults with Scoliosis." *Spine*, 33, iss. 4, 402–405.

Hartvigsen, J. and K. Christensen. "Active Lifestyle Protects Against Incident Low Back Pain in Seniors: A Population-Based 2-Year Prospective Study of 1387 Danish Twins Aged 70–100 Years." *Spine*, 32, no. 1 (January 1, 2007): 76–81.

Hartvigsen J. and K. Christensen. "Pain in the Back and Neck Are With Us Until the End: A Nationwide Interview-Based Survey of Danish 100-Year-Olds." *Spine*, 33, iss. 8 (April 15, 2008): 909–913.

Hellsten E.K. and M.A. Hanbidge. "An Economic Evaluation of Perioperative Adverse Events Associated with Spinal Surgery." *The Spine Journal*, 13, no. 44 (2013): 5.

Hellum, C. and L. Berg. "Adjacent Level Degeneration and Facet Arthopathy After Disc Prosthesis Surgery or Rehabilitation in Patients With Chronic Low Back Pain and Degenerative Disc." *Spine*, 37 (2012): 2063–2073.

Herbert J.J., S.L. Koppenhaver and B.F. Walker. "Sub-grouping Patients with Low-Back Pain: A Treatment-Based Approach to Classification, Sports Health: A Multi-Disciplinary Approach." Published online August 23, 2011.

Hestbaek, L., C. Leboeuf-Yde, M. Engberg, T. Lauritzen, N.H. Bruun and C. Manniche. 2003. "The Course of Low Back Pain in a General Population. Results from a 5-Year Prospective Study." *J Manipulative Phyiol Ther* 26(4): 213–219.

Heuscher, Zachary, MS, et al. "The Association of Self-Reported Backpack Use and Backpack Weight with Low Back Pain among College Students." *Journal of Manipulative and Physiological Therapeutics*, 33, no. 6 (July/August 2010).

Holth H.S., et al. "Physical inactivity is associated with chronic musculoskeletal complaints 11years later: Results from the Nord-Trondelag Health Study." *BMC Musculoskeletal Disorders*, 2008.

Ikeda, T., et al. "Pathomechanism of spontaneous regression of the herniated lumbar disc." *Spinal Disord*, 9, iss. 9 (April 1, 1996): 40–136.

Keeney, B.J. and D. Fulton-Kehoe. "Low-Back Pain: Healing your Aching Back. Early Predictors of Lumbar Spine Surgery after Occupational Back Injury: Results from a Prospective Study of Workers in Washington State." *Harvard Special Health Reports,* (December 12, 2012): 4.

Kline, C.M. "Working the Core, Part I: Hollowing & Bracing, Assessment, Training, and Prevention." *Focus*, July 2009.

Kline, C.M. "Working the Core, Part II: The Neuromuscular Component." *Focus*, August 2009.

Kline, C.M. "Chiropractic Approach to Lumbar Spinal Stenosis Part I." *Focus*, April 2008.

Knutson, G.A., DC, et al. "Erector Spinae and Quadratus Lumborum Muscle Endurance Tests and Supine Leg-Length Alignment Asymmetry: An Observational Study." *Journal of Manipulative and Physiological Therapeutics*, 28, no. 8 (October 2005): 575.

Kong, D.S., et al. "One-year Outcome Evaluation after Interspinous Implantation for Degenerative Spinal Stenosis with Segmental Instability." *J Korean Med Sci*, 22, (2007): 330–335.

Kruse R.A. and J. Cambron. "Spinal Manipulative Therapy for Elderly Patients with Chronic Obstructive Pulmonary Disease: A Case Series." *J Manipulative Physiol Ther*, 34 (2011): 413–417.

Lara-de-la-Fuente, R., et al. "Postoperative fibrosis after lumbar surgery." *Acta Ortop Mex*, 23, iss. 2 (May 13, 2009): 3–90.

Leboeuf-Yde, Charlotte, DC, MPH, PhD, et al. "The Nordic Back Pain Subpopulation Program: The Long-Term Outcome Pattern in Patients with Low Back Pain Treated by Chiropractors in Sweden." *Journal of Chiropractic Medicine*, 28, no. 7, (September 2005): 472.

Lis A.M., et al. "Association between sitting and occupational LBP." *European Spine Journal*, 16, no. 2 (February 2007): 283–298.

Magnusson M.L., et al. "Motor Control Learning in Chronic Low Bain Pain." *Spine*, 33, no. 3 (July 15, 2008): E532–E538.

Marshall, P.W., et al. "Extensibility of the hamstring is the best explained by mechanical components muscle behavior measures in chronic low back pain." *Electromyogr Kinesiol*, May 14, 2009.

Marshall, P. and B. Murphy, DC, PhD, et al. "The Effect of Sacroiliac Joint Manipulation On Feed-Forward Activation Times of the Deep Abdominal Musculature." *PGDip-Sci:* 196.

Martin, B.I., R.A Deyo, S.K. Mirza, J.A. Turner, B.A. Comstock, W. Hollingworth and S.D. Sullivan. "Expenditures and Health Status among Adults with Back Problems." *JAMA* 299, no. 6 (2008): 656–664.

Martin, B.I., J.A. Turner, S.K. Mirza, M.J. Lee, B.A. Comstock and R.A. Deyo. "Trends in Health Care Expenditures, Utilization, and Health Status Among US Adults With Spine Problems, 1997–2006." *Spine* 34, no. 19 (2009): 2077–2084.

Mayrand, N., et al. "Diagnosis and Management of Posttraumatic Piriformis Syndrome: A Case Study." *Journal of Manipulative and Physiological Therapeutics*, 29, no. 6, (July/August 2006).

McMorland, et al. "Manipulation or Microdiskectomy." *Journal of Chiropractic Medicine*, 33, iss. 8: 557–638.

Misaggi, B., et al. "Articular facets Syndrome; diagnostic grading and treatment options." *Spine*, May 12, 2009.

Miyamoto, G.C., et al. "The efficacy of the addition of the Pilates method over a minimal intervention in the treatment of chronic non specific low back pain: a study protocol of a randomized control trial." *Journal of Chiropractic Medicine*, 10, no. 4 (December 2011): 248–254.

Miyamoto, G.C., PT, et al. "Mechanical vs Manual Manipulation for Low Back Pain: An Observation Cohort Study." *Journal of Manipulative and Physiological Therapeutics*.

Murphy, D.R. and E.L. Hurwitz. "The Usefulness of Clinical Measures of Psychologic Factors in Patients with Spinal Pain." *J Manipulative Physiol Ther*, 34, (2011): 609–613.

Murphy, D.R., DC, et al. "A Nonsurgical Approach to the Management of Patients with Lumbar Radiculopathy Secondary to Herniated Disk: A Prospective Observational Cohort Study with Follow-Up." *Journal of Manipulative and Physiological Therapeutics*, 32, no. 9, (June 2009).

Neblett R., et al. "Quantifying the lumbar flexion-relaxation phenomenon: theory, normative data and clinical applications." *Spine*, 28, no. 13 (2003):1435–46 (ISSN: 1528-1159).

Novicoff, W.M., et al. "Does Concomitant Low Back Pain Affect Revision Total Knee Arthroplasty Outcomes." *Clin Orthp Relat Res* (May 13, 2009).

Ohtori, S., et al. "Results of Surgery for Discogenic Low Back Pain: A Randomized Study using Discogenic Discoblock for Diagnosis." *Spine*, May 15, 2009.

Owen, N., et al. "Too Much Sitting: A Novel and Important Predictor of Chronic Disease Risk?" *British Journal of Sports Medicine*, December 2008.

Owens, C., ScD, PT, et al. "Changes in Spinal Height Following Sustained Lumbar Flexion and Extension Postures: A Clinical Measure of Intervertebral Disc Hydration Using Stadiometry." *Journal of Manipulative and Physiological Therapeutics*, 31, no. 5, June 2009.

Peul, W.C., et al. "Surgery versus Prolonged Conservative Treatment for Sciatica." *The New England Journal of Medicine*, 356, no. 22 (May 31, 2007): 2245–2256.

Roelofs, P.D.D.M., et al. "Nonsteroidal Anti-inflammatory Drugs for Low Back Pain: An Updated Cochrane Review." *Spine*, 33, no. 16 (July 15, 2008): 1766–1774.

Sakai, Y., et al. "The Effects of Muscle Relaxant on the Paraspinal Muscle Blood Flow: A Randomized Controlled Trial in Patients with Chronic Low Back Pain." *Spine*, 33, iss. 6 (March 15, 2008): 581–587.

Schneider, M.J., DC, PhD, et al. "Manipulation for Low Back Pain." *Journal of Manipulative and Physiological Therapeutics*, 33, no. 3 (March/April 2010).

Schofield D.J. and R.N. Shrestha. "The Personal and National Cost of Early Retirement because of spinal Disorders: Impacts on Income, Taxes, and Governments Support Payments." *The Spine Journal*, 12, no. 12 (2012): 1111–1118.

Seidler, A., et al. "Cumulative occupational lumbar load and lumbar disc disease-result of a German control study (EPILIFT)." *BMC Musculoskelet Disord*, 10, iss. 1 (May 9, 2009): 48.

Sharma, R., M. Haas and M. Stano. "Determinants of Costs and Pain Improvement for Medical and Chiropractic Care of Low Back Pain." *J Manipulative Physiol Ther*, 32: 252–261.

Sipko, T., PT, PhD, et al. "The Occurrence of Strain Symptoms in the Lumbosacral Region and Pelvis during Pregnancy and After Childbirth." *Journal of Manipulative and Physiological Therapeutics, Stain Symptoms*, 33, no. 5 (June 2010).

Sogaard, R., et al. "Spinal Surgery Cost-Effective?" *Journal of the American Chiropractic Association, Spine*, 32 (2007): 2405–2414.

Talbot, L. "Failed back surgery syndrome." *BMJ*, 327, 7421 (October 25, 2003): 985–986.

Teodorczyk-Injeyan, J.A. PhD, et al. "Spinal Manipulative Therapy Reduces Inflammatory Cytokines but not Substance P Production in Normal Subjects." *Journal of Manipulative and Physiological Therapeutics*, 29, no. 1 (January 2006): 14.

The Chiropractic Report staff. "After the Storm–What Have We Learnt?" *The Chiropractic Report*, 4, no. 6 (November 2011): 4.

The Chiropractic Report staff. "Best Treatment for Neck Pain." *The Chiropractic Report*, 26, no. 26 (March 2012): 4.

The Chiropractic Report staff. "CAM or Mainstream? Where is the Chiropractic Profession, Why is this Important?" *The Chiropractic Report*, 23, no. 1 (January 2009): 5.

The Chiropractic Report staff. "Changed Medical and Surgical Attitudes. Working with Chiropractors in Managing Spine Pain Patients." *The Chiropractic Report*, 27, no. 3 (May 2013): 1–8.

The Chiropractic Report staff. "Chiropractic Managements of Children and Infants." *The Chiropractic Report*, 23, no. 4 (July 2009).

The Chiropractic Report staff. "Cost-Effectiveness Revisited, A New Report from US Health Economists." *The Chiropractic Report*, 23, no. 6 (November 2009): 1–8.

The Chiropractic Report staff. "Current Status of the Profession." *The Chiropractic Report*, 27, no. 2 (March 2013).

The Chiropractic Report staff. "Management of Patients with Back Pain, The New Medical and Chiropractic Consensus." *The Chiropractic Report*, 23, no. 5 (September 2009): 1–8.

The Chiropractic Report staff. "Market Identity of the Profession, WFC, Palmer College, World Spine Day, World Spine Care." *The Chiropractic Report*, 27, no. 1 (January 2013): 5.

The Chiropractic Report staff. "New Best Practices for Chiropractic, Patient-Centered vs. Payer-Centered Care." *The Chiropractic Report*, 23, no. 2 (March 2009).

The Chiropractic Report staff. "Supermarket of Science for Chronic Back Pain." *The Chiropractic Report*, 22, no. 3 (May 2008): 1–8.

The Chiropractic Report staff. "The Art of Writing Letters and Reports." *The Chiropractic Report*, 26, no.1 (January 2012): 4–5.

The Chiropractic Report staff. "The Chiropractic Profession, Basic Facts, Independent Evaluations, Common Questions Answered." *The Chiropractic Report*, 22, no. 5 (September 2008): 1–8.

The Chiropractic Report staff. "The Road to Integration, WFC's Montreal Congress Report on Progress." *The Chiropractic Report*, 23, no. 3 (May 2009): 4.

Thomas J.S. and C.R. France. "Pain-Related Fear Is Associated With Avoidance of Spinal Motion During Recovery From Low Back Pain." *Spine*, 32, iss. 16 (July 15, 2007): E460–E466.

Triano, J.J., et al. "What Constitutes Evidence for Best Practice?" *J Manipulative Physiol Ther*, 31 (2008): 637–643.

Turner, J.A. and G. Franklin. "ISSLS Prize Winner: Early Predictors of Chronic Work Disability: A Prospective, Population–Based Study of Workers with Back Injuries." *Spine*, 33, no. 25 (2008): 4, 2809–2818.

Van Vugt, R.M., et al. "Antioxidant intervention in rheumatoid arthritis: results of an open pilot study." *Clinical Rheumatology*, 27, no. 6 (June 2008): 771–775.

Womersley, L., MSc and S. May, BSc. "Sitting Posture of Subjects with Postural Backache." *JMPT* (March/April 2006): 213.

LIST OF VIDEOS

Video 1: Finding Neutral (http://dukechironyc.com/cumulus/videos/10/video-1-finding-neutral/)

Video 2: Kneeling to Standing Abdominal Bracing (http://dukechironyc.com/cumulus/videos/11/video-2-kneeling-to-standing-abdominal-bracing/)

Video 3: Sky Reaches (http://dukechironyc.com/cumulus/videos/112/video-3-sky-reaches/)

Video 4: Swimmer (http://dukechironyc.com/cumulus/videos/17/video-4-swimmer/)

Video 5: Backstroke (http://dukechironyc.com/cumulus/videos/18/video-5-backstroke/)

Video 6: Angels (http://dukechironyc.com/cumulus/videos/19/video-6-angels/)

Video 7: Golf Twists (http://dukechironyc.com/cumulus/videos/20/video-7-golf-twists/)

Video 8: Pelvic Twist (http://dukechironyc.com/cumulus/videos/21/video-8-pelvic-twists/)

Video 9: Pelvic Clocks (http://dukechironyc.com/cumulus/videos/22/video-9-pelvic-clocks/)

Video 10: Pelvic Thrust (http://dukechironyc.com/cumulus/videos/23/video-10-pelvic-thrust/)

Video 11: Hip Gyro (http://dukechironyc.com/cumulus/videos/24/video-11-hip-gyro/)

Video 12: Lunge and Reach (http://dukechironyc.com/cumulus/videos/25/video-12-lunge-and-reach/)

Video 13: Bowling (http://dukechironyc.com/cumulus/videos/26/video-13-bowling/)

Video 14: Hacky Sack (http://dukechironyc.com/cumulus/videos/27/video-14-hacky-sack/)

Video 15: Counter Traction (http://dukechironyc.com/cumulus/videos/28/video-15-counter-traction/)

Video 16: Leg Swings (http://dukechironyc.com/cumulus/videos/29/video-16-leg-swings/)

Video 17: Diagonal Leg Swings (http://dukechironyc.com/cumulus/videos/30/video-17-diagonal-leg-swings/)

Video 18: Descending Hip Drops (http://dukechironyc.com/cumulus/videos/113/video-18-descending-hip-drops/)

Video 19: Pelvic Release (http://dukechironyc.com/cumulus/videos/33/video-19-pelvic-release/)

Video 20: Back Bridges (http://dukechironyc.com/cumulus/videos/34/video-20-back-bridges/)

Video 21: Marching Bridge (http://dukechironyc.com/cumulus/videos/35/video-21-marching-bridge/)

Video 22: Knee Hugs Bridge (http://dukechironyc.com/cumulus/videos/36/video-22-knee-hugs-bridge/)

Video 23: Dynamic Hamstrings (http://dukechironyc.com/cumulus/videos/37/video-23-dynamic-hamstrings/)

Video 24: Hip Openers (http://dukechironyc.com/cumulus/videos/38/video-24-hip-openers/)

Video 25: Windshield Wipers (http://dukechironyc.com/cumulus/videos/39/video-25-windshield-wipers/)

Video 26: Clam Shell (http://dukechironyc.com/cumulus/videos/40/video-26-clam-shell/)

Video 27: Dynamic Hip Flexors (http://dukechironyc.com/cumulus/videos/114/video-27-dynamic-hip-flexors)

Video 28: Open Book (http://dukechironyc.com/cumulus/videos/42/video-28-open-book/)

Video 29: Ab Curls (http://dukechironyc.com/cumulus/videos/43/video-29-ab-curls/)

Video 30: Front Plank (http://dukechironyc.com/cumulus/videos/44/video-30-front-plank/)

Video 31: Side Bridges (http://dukechironyc.com/cumulus/videos/45/video-31-side-bridges/)

Video 32: Reach-Backs (http://dukechironyc.com/cumulus/videos/47/video-32-reach-backs/)

Video 33: Point and Reach (http://dukechironyc.com/cumulus/videos/48/video-33-point-and-reach/)

Video 34: Cat and Cow (http://dukechironyc.com/cumulus/videos/49/video-34-cat-and-cow/)

Video 35: Seated Sky Reaches (http://dukechironyc.com/cumulus/videos/50/video-35-seated-sky-reaches/)

Video 36: Seated Angels (http://dukechironyc.com/cumulus/videos/51/video-36-seated-angels/)

Video 37: Seated Back Arching (http://dukechironyc.com/cumulus/videos/52/video-37-seated-back-arching/)

Video 38: Seated Side Bends (http://dukechironyc.com/cumulus/videos/53/video-38-seated-side-bends/)

Video 39: Seated Golf Twists (http://dukechironyc.com/cumulus/videos/54/video-39-seated-golf-twists/)

Video 40: Seated Posture Reset (http://dukechironyc.com/cumulus/videos/55/video-40-seated-posture-reset/)

Video 41: Seated Hip Closers and Openers (http://dukechironyc.com/cumulus/videos/56/video-41-seated-hip-closers-and-openers/)

Video 42: Seated Back Traction (http://dukechironyc.com/cumulus/videos/58/video-42-seated-back-traction/)

Video 43: Standing Back Arch (http://dukechironyc.com/cumulus/videos/59/video-43-standing-back-arch/)

Video 44: Lunge and Reach (http://dukechironyc.com/cumulus/videos/60/video-44-lunge-and-reach/)

Video 45: Diving Archer (http://dukechironyc.com/cumulus/videos/61/video-45-diving-and-archer/)

Video 46: Standing Pelvic Thrusts (http://dukechironyc.com/cumulus/videos/62/video-46-standing-pelvic-twist/)

Video 47: Golf Twists (http://dukechironyc.com/cumulus/videos/63/video-47-golf-twists/)

Video 48: Standing Pelvic Twists (http://dukechironyc.com/cumulus/videos/64/video-48-standing-pelvic-twists/)

Video 49: Standing Pelvic Clocks (http://dukechironyc.com/cumulus/videos/66/video-49-standing-pelvic-clocks/)

Video 50: Hacky Sack (http://dukechironyc.com/cumulus/videos/67/video-50-hacky-sack/)

Video 51: Counter Traction (http://dukechironyc.com/cumulus/videos/68/video-51-counter-traction/)

Video 52: Recumbent Pelvic Tilts (http://dukechironyc.com/cumulus/videos/69/video-52-recumbent-pelvic-tilts/)

Video 53: Side Stretch (http://dukechironyc.com/cumulus/videos/70/video-53-side-stretch/)

Video 54: Lunge Stretch (http://dukechironyc.com/cumulus/videos/71/video-54-lunge-stretch/)

Video 55: Hip Rotator Stretch (http://dukechironyc.com/cumulus/videos/72/video-55-hip-rotator-stretch/)

Video 56: Hamstring Stretch (http://dukechironyc.com/cumulus/videos/73/video-56-hamstring-stretch/)

Video 57: Full Spine Stretch (http://dukechironyc.com/cumulus/videos/74/video-57-full-spine-stretch/)

Video 58: Hanging Thigh Stretch (http://dukechironyc.com/cumulus/videos/75/video-58-hanging-thigh-stretch/)

Video 59: Lunge on Stool Stretch (http://dukechironyc.com/cumulus/videos/76/video-59-lunge-on-stool-stretch/)

Video 60: Standing Lunge Stretch (http://dukechironyc.com/cumulus/videos/77/video-60-standing-lunge-stretch/)

Video 61: Side Lying Hip Rotator Stretch (http://dukechironyc.com/cumulus/videos/78/video-61-side-lying-hp-rotator-stretch/)

Video 62: Front Plank (http://dukechironyc.com/cumulus/videos/79/video-62-front-plank/)

Video 63: Half Plank (http://dukechironyc.com/cumulus/videos/80/video-63-half-plank/)

Video 64: Single Leg Back Bridge (http://dukechironyc.com/cumulus/videos/81/video-64-single-leg-back-bridge/)

Video 65: Back Bridge Using Two Legs (http://dukechironyc.com/cumulus/videos/82/video-65-back-bridge-using-two-legs/)

Video 66: Side Bridge (http://dukechironyc.com/cumulus/videos/83/video-66-side-bridge/)

Video 67: Half-Side Bridge (http://dukechironyc.com/cumulus/videos/84/video-67-half-side-bridge/)

Video 68: Straight Leg Torso Lift (http://dukechironyc.com/cumulus/videos/85/video-68-straight-leg-torso-lift/)

Video 69: Ab Curls–Elbows Up (http://dukechironyc.com/cumulus/videos/86/video-69-ab-curls-elbows-up/)

Video 70: Ab Curls–Hand on Head (http://dukechironyc.com/cumulus/videos/87/video-70-ab-curls-hand-on-head/)

Video 71: Point and Reach (http://dukechironyc.com/cumulus/videos/88/video-71-point-and-reach/)

Video 72: Point and Reach–Elbow Knee (http://dukechironyc.com/cumulus/videos/90/video-72-point-and-reach-elbow-knee/)

Video 73: Cat/Cow (http://dukechironyc.com/cumulus/videos/91/video-73-cat-cow/)

Video 74: Lower Back Belt (http://dukechironyc.com/cumulus/videos/92/video-74-lower-back-belt/)

Video 75: Pelvic Shift (http://dukechironyc.com/cumulus/videos/93/video-75-pelvic-shift/)

Video 76A: Lying Sciatica Flossing (http://dukechironyc.com/cumulus/videos/94/video-76a-lieing-sciatica-flossing/)

Video 76B: Seated Sciatica Flossing (http://dukechironyc.com/cumulus/videos/115/video-76b-seated-sciatica-flossing/)

Video 77: Lower Back Belt (http://dukechironyc.com/cumulus/videos/96/video-77-lower-back-belt/)

Video 78: Facet Decompression Stretch (http://dukechironyc.com/cumulus/videos/97/video-78-facet-decompression-stretch/)

Video 79: Three-way Calf Stretch (http://dukechironyc.com/cumulus/videos/98/video-79-three-way-calf-stretch/)

Video 80: Foam Roller (http://dukechironyc.com/cumulus/videos/116/video-80-foam-roller/)

Video 81: Foam Roller for Piriformis (http://dukechironyc.com/cumulus/videos/100/video-81-foam-roller-for-piriformis/)

Video 82: Lying Pelvic Thrusts (http://dukechironyc.com/cumulus/videos/101/video-82-lying-pelvic-thrusts/)

Video 83: 3 Way Prayer Pose (http://dukechironyc.com/cumulus/videos/102/video-83-3-way-prayer-pose/)

Video 84: Upper Quadriceps Stretch (http://dukechironyc.com/cumulus/videos/103/video-84-upper-quadriceps-stretch/)

Video 85: Supine Knee to Chest (http://dukechironyc.com/cumulus/videos/104/video-85-supine-knee-to-chest/)

Video 86: Abdominal Punch (http://dukechironyc.com/cumulus/videos/105/video-86-abdominal-punch/)

Video 87: Double Knee to Chest (http://dukechironyc.com/cumulus/videos/106/video-87-double-knee-to-chest/)

Index

synovial fluid 48

T

TFL stretch 215
tibialis posterior 180
twisting 28
two-leg back bridge 137

U

upper body training
   overhead presses 205
   seated rows 205
upper quadriceps stretch 217

V

vertebroplasty 229

W

warrior one pose 188
water 256
weight lifting.
   See upper-body training
wheel or upward bow (urdhva dhanursana) 192
windshield wipers 71
worker's compensation 171

Y

yoga 94, 184–196
  poses
    backbend 191
    beneficial to back health 186–189
    bow (dhanurasana) 190
    cat and cow 80, 111, 144, 186
    cobra
      modified 101, 109
      variation 187
    detrimental to back health 190–197
    diving archer 94
    downward dog 189
    front bend 193
    headstand (sirasana) 197
    locust (salabhasana) 192
    plank
      front 76, 134
      half 135
    plow (halasana) 195
    prayer 238, 247
    reclining hero (supta virasana) 198
    seated forward bend (paschimottansana) 194
    shoulder stand (sarvangasana) 196
    spinal twist (ardha matsyendrasana) 187
    standing forward bend (uttanasana) 194
    warrior one 188
    wheel or upward bow (urdhva dhanursana) 192

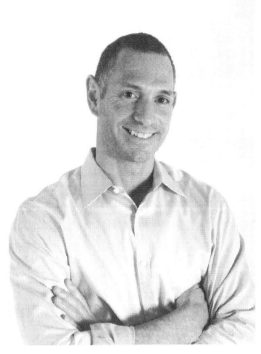

DR. SCOTT G. DUKE is a graduate of the New York College of Chiropractic. He received his Bachelor of Science in Kinesiology from the University of Maryland, College Park in 1985, and he received an additional Bachelor of Science in Human Anatomy from the National College of Chiropractic, Chicago, Illinois in 1987, where he also worked as a research scientist in the Spinal Ergonomics and Biomechanics Laboratory. He earned his Doctorate in Chiropractic from the New York College of Chiropractic, Long Island, New York in 1990. In 1992, he became a chiropractic sports physician and earned Diplomate status in sports medicine from the American Chiropractic Board of Sports Physicians. He is an expert in the field of sports science and spinal rehabilitation, and has been a strength and conditioning specialist certified by the National Strength and Conditioning Association since 1986.

Dr. Duke specializes in the treatment of soft tissue injuries caused by daily microtrauma and he was an educator on the revolutionary Active Release Technique (ART). He uses a variety of techniques and exercises in his evaluation and treatment process including instrument assisted soft tissue manipulation with the Graston Technique, neuromuscular re-education and therapeutic movement oriented exercises. His background with the Titleist Golf Performance Institute, in addition to his expertise in medicine, kinesiology and biomechanics, enables him to not only effectively treat his patients, but to also enhance their athletic performance.

Current medical staff appointments and past experiences include: Team USA United States Olympic Committees National Medical Network Physician; chiropractic sports physician for a team of elite and professional runners, New York Road Runners; Physician Team Captain for the ING NYC Marathon and the NYC Triathlon since 1995; strength and conditioning coach for the Chicago Blackhawks NHL hockey team from 1986–1988; sports chiropractor at the United States Olympic Games of 1992, in Atlanta, Georgia, and at the United States Olympic Training Center (USOTC), in Colorado Springs, Colorado, in 1997; and chiropractic sports physician for the National and World Championships for Competitive Aerobics in 1995.

Dr. Duke lectures professionally and academically in addition to multiple broadcast appearances. He has published numerous scientific papers on muscle power development through plyometric training and its use in enhancing athletic performance. He is a co-creator of the Apple app called W.E.RUN. It is designed to aid coaches train athletes and help individuals who train for endurance sports dynamically warm up—specifically for swimming, biking, running and triathlons. He is the author of Crunch Health Club's *Perfect Posture* and the Bally Health Club's flexibility and stretching manual. Dr. Duke has also been published in *Self, Allure, Men's Health, Runner's World, New York Runner, Competitor* and many other magazines and online resources. More information about Dr. Duke can be found at the following sites: www.dukechironyc.com, www.twitter.com/drscottduke, and www.facebook.com/dukechiropractic.

Dr. Scott Duke DC DACBSP CSCS
212-481-0066
9 East 38th Street, 9th floor
New York City, New York 10016

Made in the USA
Lexington, KY
10 July 2014